Breath Odors

Nir Sterer · Mel Rosenberg

Breath Odors

Origin, Diagnosis, and Management

Second Edition

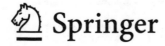 Springer

Nir Sterer
Department of Prosthodontics,
Goldschleger School of Dental Medicine
Sackler Faculty of Medicine, Tel Aviv
University
Tel Aviv
Israel

Mel Rosenberg
Department of Clinical Microbiology
and Immunology
Sackler Faculty of Medicine, Tel Aviv
University
Tel Aviv
Israel

ISBN 978-3-030-44733-5   ISBN 978-3-030-44731-1   (eBook)
https://doi.org/10.1007/978-3-030-44731-1

This Springer imprint is published by the registered company Springer Nature Switzerland AG
The registered company address is: Gewerbestrasse 11, 6330 Cham, Switzerland

Contents

Introduction

Breath odor is a common condition affecting those who have it, and those in their proximity. Until the 1980s, most research was carried out at private companies (mainly those producing mouthwash and those testing it) who tended to publish little and protect as much of their "know-how" as possible. There were only a few scientists working on this subject in isolated university laboratories, often separated by thousands of kilometers.

However, the past three decades have seen this subject spawn a scientific community, with a society (ISBOR, the International Society for Breath Odor Research), international conferences and a successful international journal (The Journal of Breath Research, IOP Publishing). The growing body of research in the field of bad breath has managed to shed light on some of the main questions while others still remain open.

It is clear that in the vast majority (some 85–90%) of the cases breath odors derives from the oral cavity itself. Other sources may include nasopharyngeal or upper respiratory conditions, metabolic disorders, systemic diseases, and other external sources. In the oral cavity, most of the odor is due to putrefactive microbial activity. It is not yet clear, however, whether the bacteria responsible for the odor are a specific group of only a few species or rather hundreds of types, and to what extent they vary from individual to individual. In vitro, odor is not elaborated except under anaerobic conditions, yet it is not clear

whether the bacteria involved are obligate anaerobes. It is not known whether the odor is produced independently by individual species or due to cooperation (e.g., between Gram-positive species producing glycosidases and Gram-negative anaerobes). Finally, is *Solobacterium moorei* a causative bacterium in the odor process, or rather merely present in the mouths of those with malodor?

There is a wide consensus that the posterior area of the tongue dorsum is the major site of malodor production. Other sites in the oral cavity may be involved as well (e.g., interdental plaque and inflamed pockets). However, the typical odor from the back of the tongue is quite different in quality as compared with interdental or subgingival odor, as well as denture odor. This difference in odor character between the various sites is not yet understood. Whether these dissimilarities are a function of different bacterial types involved at the various sites, or rather the different substrate available for degradation? Further, although many (but not all) studies link tongue coating with malodor, it is not clear to what extent differences in tongue morphologies (e.g., fissured tongue) contribute to observed differences in odor.

It is commonly held that during the day, odor is worst when our mouth dries out (especially upon awakening). Is this because the odors evaporate more readily from the drying mucosal surfaces or because of microbial accumulation in the absence of the cleansing and/or antibacterial

© Springer Nature Switzerland AG 2020
N. Sterer, M. Rosenberg, *Breath Odors*, https://doi.org/10.1007/978-3-030-44731-1_1

effects of saliva? To what extent is drying saliva a substrate for malodor production in the mouth? Some studies suggest that clinical xerostomia does not predispose to oral malodor. Is this because of the acidic pH, different microbiota, or other reasons?

It is evident that volatile sulfides, in particular, hydrogen sulfide and methyl mercaptan can be readily detected in breath, and their levels correlate with breath odor. Does this mean that they are the only gases responsible for the breath odor bouquet? Some researchers are of the opinion that this is the case, while others do not. Both sulfide gases are significantly correlated with odor judge scores in many studies, regardless of the measuring techniques (e.g., GC, halimeter, OralChroma). It should be kept in mind, however, that hydrogen sulfide and methyl mercaptan are associated with many other types of microbial odors (e.g., feces, sewage, animal waste, putrefying foods) that are dissimilar to breath odors. Furthermore, one would still have to account for the variation in odor types for various kinds of oral malodor.

As stated above, breath odor is often worst upon awakening. In the absence of poor oral hygiene or other pathological factors, morning breath might thus be considered a normal human characteristic, and is often termed physiological halitosis. However, there are no studies available to determine whether people with healthy dentition and gums, with little or non-tongue coating, who practice excellent daily oral hygiene, should have any breath odor at all upon awakening? So is morning breath in the absence of periodontal inflammation or disease "physiological bad breath," as some researchers have described it or not?

People with bad breath who are completely unaware that they suffer from the problem are commonly encountered by us all. However, the reason for this is not yet clear. Is it because of psychological habituation, physiological adaptation, our physical inability to breathe in through our nose what we breathe out through our mouth? There are thus millions of people with bad breath who do not know, and millions of others without bad breath who are sure they do. This is com-

pounded by the reticence of others (even family members) to alert someone that they suffer from breath odor.

Most of the population tend to worry to varying degrees about whether their breath is fine or not. However, a portion of the population (some 1–2% of the adult population) worries a lot. For them it is a continuous preoccupation. There are some potential factors that lead people to be overly concerned: aggressive advertising, foul smelling tonsillar stones (i.e., tonsilloliths), having been told once in the past, having parents with bad breath, bad taste, etc. Why do these exaggerated worries persist and ruin people's quality of life? Should an exaggerated concern of bad breath be considered a continuous spectrum (according to the original definition of halitophobia), or be separated into two dichotomous groups, the first of which is amenable to treatment (i.e., "pseudo-halitosis")? How close is the unnecessary worry of having body odor to other concerns of abnormal body parts and functions? Should the psychiatric definition of "body dysmorphic disorder" be extended to include worries about smells, for example? To what extent can excessive worries of having bad breath be dealt with by psychological counseling and medication? These are all questions under current discussion.

Further, we are often asked about the possibility of "inheriting" bad breath. This could take two forms, the first inheriting genes which predispose to bad breath (e.g., related perhaps to the immune system, tooth, tongue, and nose anatomy), the second "inheriting" odor-producing bacterial species from our parents (the same way that caries-producing strains are inherited). Little research has been done in this area.

There is also a controversy surrounding the role of the tonsils in breath odor. Most researchers think they play only a minor role, while there are others who think that they are important. However, there are few studies to support the latter contention. Further, subjects with tonsilloliths often worry about bad breath because of the odor of the tonsil stones, but there is little information on their contribution to the overall halitosis whilst in the crypts.

Finally, we know little about the potentially causal relationship between malodorous gases in the mouth and periodontal disease. It appears that bad breath is more directly related to current signs of gingival bleeding and inflammation indices than pocket status or plaque index. Given the ample data showing that malodorous gases, such as hydrogen sulfide, are highly toxic to soft tissue, might one assume that these microbial gases help promote cell death and the advance of the disease. It is also unclear to what extent the putrefaction on the tongue impacts the health of the periodontium.

Odor judge scoring is another issue that requires future scrutiny. With all the limitations of using human judges, they are still considered the gold standard of breath testing. Yet, few studies are available comparing the scoring of multiple judges. Training sessions conducted at Prof. John Greenman's laboratory in Bristol teach us that judges differ in their abilities to discriminate various odor molecules, as well as the concentrations of a given stimulant. Will training sessions (or kits) help calibrate researchers worldwide? Hopefully reliable instruments able to detect low concentrations of non-sulfide gases (e.g. indole, skatole, cadaverine, and putrescine), will become available, allowing researchers to better ascertain their role in oral malodor, and to come up with instrumental assessments that more closely resemble odor judge scores.

The main goal of the present textbook is to describe, summarize, and elaborate on the growing body of knowledge accumulated over the years in both research and clinical aspects of the field of breath odors. What we have learned, and what still remains to be learnt.

Breath Odors of Oral Origin (Oral Malodor)

2

Contents

Breath odors or halitosis denotes any type of disagreeable scent felt on a person's breath during exhalation and speech. These odors have many different causes and may originate from various locations such as the oral cavity, tonsils, nasal cavity, upper respiratory tract, and the lungs.

According to research performed in several multidisciplinary breath clinics (involving professionals from various fields: dentistry, E.N.T., internal medicine, and psychology) in various centers, some 85–90% of breath odors originate from within the oral cavity itself (Table 2.1). This condition in which the malodor originates from the mouth is commonly known as oral malodor (also termed: *Fetor oris* or *Feotor ex ora*) and will be discussed in the present chapter (for extraoral sources see Chaps. 5–7).

The potential loci for malodor production within the oral cavity include the posterior portion of tongue's dorsum, subgingival areas (e.g., periodontal pockets and interdental spaces),

faulty restorations (e.g., leaking crowns and bridges), dental implants, dentures, and appliances. Furthermore, transient oral dryness brought about by a temporary reduction in saliva flow plays an important part in promoting this condition.

Oral malodor is measured directly by human odor judges, or by adjunct measurements, such as the levels of volatile sulfide compounds (VSC) within the oral cavity (for further details, see Chap. 8).

2.1 Oral Malodor and the Tongue

The data presented in Table 2.1 clearly demonstrate that the tongue is by far the most common source for malodor production within the oral cavity. This was first suggested by Grapp in 1933. The posterior portion of the tongue's dorsum, where most malodor originates, is often covered by a layer of debris comprising of cellular (bacteria, desquamated epithelial cell, white blood cells), and noncellular components (especially proteins from saliva, postnasal and gingival secretions). This layer termed "tongue coating" (Fig. 2.1) may vary in size, thickness, and color among and within different individuals

depending on oral activity (e.g., eating, drinking, smoking), oral hygiene, and oral health-related parameters (e.g., presence of periodontal disease; Yaegaki and Sanada 1992a, b).

Over the last four decades, various measuring techniques have been suggested for tongue

Table 2.1 Distribution of breath odor origins in subjects attending multidisciplinary clinics

References	Patients population	Confirmed breath odor problem	
Quirynen et al. (2009)	$N = 2000$ (1078 F) Age 2–90 years (39.2 ± 14.2)	$N = 1687$ (84.3%)	
		Oral causes $N = 1515$ (89.8%)	Non-oral causes $N = 97$ (5.7%)
		Tongue coating (TC) $N = 868$ (51.4%) Gingivitis (G) $N = 75$ (4.4%) Periodontitis (P) $N = 148$ (8.7%) Combination (TC/G/P) $N = 363$ (21.5%) Xerostomia $N = 50$ (2.9%) Dental $N = 7$ (0.4%) Candida $N = 4$ (0.2%)	ENT Tonsillitis $N = 14$ (0.8%) Rhinitis $N = 11$ (0.6%) Sinusitis $N = 4$ (0.2%) Nose obstruction $N = 8$ (0.4%) Extra oral: GI tract $N = 26$ (1.5%) TMAU $N = 1$ (0.05%) Systemic $N = 5$ (0.2%) Medication $N = 2$ (0.1%) Hormonal $N = 2$ (0.1%) Diet $N = 9$ (0.5%) Unknown $N = 15$ (0.8%)
		Oral–non-oral combination $N = 75$ (4.3%)	
		ENT + Oral: $N = 42$ (2.4%) GI + Oral: $N = 33$ (1.9%)	
Delanghe et al. (1996)	$N = 260$ (135 F) Age 2–77 years (36 ± 13.5)	$N = 246$ (94.6%)	
		Oral causes $N = 225$ (91.4%)	Non-oral causes $N = 21$ (8.5%)
		Tongue coating $N = 92$ (37.3%) Gingivitis $N = 70$ (28.4%) Periodontitis $N = 63$ (25.6%)	ENT: Chr. Tonsillitis $N = 15$ (6%) Chr. Sinusitis $N = 4$ (1.6%) Foreign bodies $N = 1$ (0.4%) Rhinitis $N = 1$ (0.4%)

Table 2.1 (continued)

References	Patients population	Confirmed breath odor problem	
Seemann et al. (2006)	$N = 407$ (204 F) Age 6–76 years (41.5 ± 13.8)	$N = 293$ (72%)	
		Oral causes $N = 272$ (92.7%)	Non-oral causes $N = 22$ (7.3%)
		Tongue coating ("physiologic") $N = 175$ (59.7%) "Pathologic" $N = 97$ (33%): Periodontitis $n = 80$ (27.3%) Gingival hyperplasia $n = 10$ (3.4%) Faulty restorations $n = 6$ (2%)	ENT: Chr. Tonsillitis $N = 15$ (5.1%) Chr. Sinusitis $N = 2$ (0.6%) Foreign bodies $N = 2$ (0.6%) Systemic: Diabetes $N = 2$ (0.6%) Smokers breath $N = 3$ (1%)
Zürcher and Filippi (2012)	$N = 451$ (218 F) Age 6–83 years (mean age 43.7)	$N = 373$ (82.7%)	
		Oral causes $N = 359$ (96.2%)	Non-oral causes $N = 14$ (3.8%)
		Tongue coating $N = 382$ (84.7%) Periodontitis $N = 87$ (19.3%) Gingivitis $N = 69$ (15.3%)	ENT $N = 11$ (2.9%) GI $N = 3$ (0.8%)

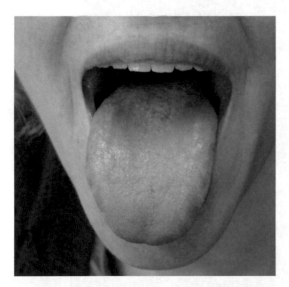

Fig. 2.1 Typical photo of a mild tongue coating covering the posterior third of the tongue dorsum

coating evaluation and quantification taking into account various parameters such as coating thickness, coating area, and discoloration. Some of these methods are summarized in Table 2.2.

Table 2.2 Tongue coating measurements

References	Score	Description
Gross et al. (1975)	0	No coating
	1	Slight coating
	2	Moderate coating
	3	Heavy coating
Yaegaki and Sanada (1992a)	Wet weight (mg)	Scraping off and weighing the tongue coating.
Miyazaki et al. (1995)	0	None visible
	1	<1/3 tongue dorsum surface covered
	2	<2/3 tongue dorsum surface covered
	3	>2/3 tongue dorsum surface covered
Mantilla Gomez et al. (2001)	*Discoloration*	
	0	Pink
	1	White
	2	Yellow/light brown
	3	Brown
	4	Black
	Thickness	
	0	No coating
	1	Light-thin coating
	2	Heavy-thick coating

(continued)

Table 2.2 (continued)

References	Score	Description
Oho et al. (2001)	*Area*	Area score × thickness score = tongue coating (range 0–6)
	0	No tongue coating
	1	<1/3 tongue dorsum surface covered
	2	1/3–2/3 tongue dorsum surface covered
	3	>2/3 tongue dorsum surface covered
	Thickness	
	0	No tongue coating
	1	Thin tongue coating (papillae visible)
	2	Thick tongue coating (papillae invisible)
Winkel et al. (2003)	(Six areas grid)	Tongue dorsum is divided into six areas (i.e., three posterior and three anterior)
	Coating	
	0	No coating
	1	Light coating
	2	Severe coating
	Discoloration	
	0	No discoloration
	1	Light discoloration
	2	Severe discoloration
		Score is calculated by adding all six scores (range 0–12)
Kim et al. (2009)	Tongue coating area	Calculated from digital images obtained by the digital tongue imaging system (DTIS)
Amou et al. (2014)	0	Not visible
	1	<1/3 covered with thin coating
	2	<2/3 thin coating or <1/3 thick coating
	3	>2/3 thin coating or >1/3 thick coating
	4	>2/3 covered with thick coating
Lee et al. (2016)	Integrated fluorescence (IF) score	Calculated by multiplying tongue coating red fluorescence (RF) intensity and area. (IF = RF intensity × RF area)

Large epidemiological studies on the prevalence of oral malodor and its related parameters in the general population have been conducted in Japan (Miyazaki et al. 1995), China (Liu et al. 2006), and Switzerland (Bornstein et al. 2009). Significant associations have been reported comparing oral malodor with the level of tongue coating (Table 2.3). Furthermore, the level of

Table 2.3 Correlations among malodor-related parameters

References	Malodor-related parameters	Correlations
Miyazaki et al. (1995) ($n = 2672$)		*Spearman correlation*
	Tongue coating[a] vs. sulfide monitor	$r = 0.44^*$–0.57^*
	Periodontal condition[b] vs. sulfide monitor	$r = 0.34^*$–0.58^*
	Plaque index[e] vs. sulfide monitor	$r = 0.13^*$–0.31^* ($^*p < 0.001$)
Liu et al. (2006) ($n = 2000$)		*Pearson correlation*
	Tongue coating[a] vs. sulfide monitor	$r = 0.15^*$–0.24^*
	Periodontal condition[d] vs. sulfide monitor:	
	Calculus	$r = 0.04^{NS}$–0.21^*
	Pocket depth	$r = 0.02^{NS}$–0.25^*
	Bleeding index	$r = 0.02^{NS}$–0.30^*
	Plaque index[c] vs. sulfide monitor	$r = 0.08^{NS}$–0.21^*
	Tongue coating1 vs. odor judge	$r = 0.20^*$–0.31^*
	Periodontal condition[d] vs. odor judge	
	Calculus	$r = 0.20^*$–0.29^*
	Pocket depth	$r = 0.17^*$–0.31^*
	Bleeding index	$r = 0.12^*$–0.22^*
	Plaque index[c] vs. odor judge	$r = 0.15^*$–0.26^* (^{NS}–nonsignificant, $^*p < 0.01$)
Bornstein et al. (2009) ($n = 419$)		*Linear regression*
	Tongue coating[e] vs. sulfide monitor	4.29
	Tongue coating[e] vs. odor judge	2.35
	Periodontal condition[d] vs. odor judge	2.45

Table 2.3 (continued)

References	Malodor-related parameters	Correlations
Amou et al. (2014) ($n = 94$)		*Spearman correlation*
	Tongue coating[f] vs. sulfide levels	$r = 0.27; p < 0.01$
	Tongue coating[f] vs. odor judge	$r = 0.33; p < 0.01$
Lee et al. (2016) ($n = 103$)		*Spearman correlation*
	Tongue coating[g] vs. sulfide levels	$r = 0.49; p < 0.01$
	Tongue coating[g] vs. odor judge	$r = 0.54; p < 0.01$

[a]Tongue coating area: 0 = none, 1 = less than 1/3, 2 = less than 2/3, 3 = more than 2/3
[b]According to WHO guidelines (CPITN)
[c]Silness and Löe 1964
[d]Periodontal screening index (PSI)
[e]0 = no coating, 1 = light coating (10%), 2 = moderate (10–50%), 3 = severe (>50%)
[f]Tongue coating area and thickness: 0 = not visible, 1 = <1/3 thin, 2 = <2/3 thin or <1/3 thick, 3 = >2/3 thin or >1/3 thick, 4 = >2/3 thick
[g]Tongue coating integrated fluorescence (IF) score

malodor-related compounds (e.g., sulfide-containing compounds) produced on the posterior portion of the tongue dorsum was highly correlated with the overall mouth odor as measured by a human odor judge ($r = 0.77$, $p < 0.01$), as well as volatile sulfide levels ($r = 0.63, p < 0.01$) (Morita et al. 2001).

Various studies comparing the tongue parameters of subjects with and without oral malodor showed that subjects with oral malodor had significantly greater tongue coating as compared with the no malodor controls (Haraszthy et al. 2007; Oho et al. 2001; Washio et al. 2005). Furthermore, mechanical removal of tongue coating results in a substantial decrease in oral malodor and its components (Yaegaki and Sanada 1992a). Research done by Tonzetich and Ng (1976) showed that tongue brushing was very effective in reducing over 70% of the volatile sulfides as compared with about 30% reduction that resulted from tooth brushing.

Some researchers suggested that postnasal drip may contribute to oral malodor formation by supplying additional mucinous substrate to the back of the tongue. In fact, one study showed

increased levels of the volatile sulfide compound methyl mercaptan in subjects with allergic rhinitis that is the main cause of postnasal drip (Avincsal et al. 2016).

Although the etiology for tongue coating formation is not entirely understood, some evidence have suggested the possible influence of genetic factors. For example, in a study conducted on 51 pairs of twins, the concordance rates for the presence of tongue coating among identical twins were 67% as compared with only 11% among fraternal twins (Bretz et al. 2011).

Tongue coating samples can be obtained by scraping the posterior portion of the tongue's dorsum using wooden spatula, plastic spoons, tooth brushes, swabs, or a gauze pads (Grapp 1933). These samples very often release a putrid malodor very similar in character to oral malodor. Sampling the tongue coating using a plastic spoon (i.e., "spoon test"; (Rosenberg 1996) and scoring the malodor emanating from the spoon yielded highly significant associations with the oral malodor scores (i.e., odor judge) as well as other oral malodor-related parameters (Table 2.4).

2.2 Oral Malodor, Gingival Health, and Periodontal Disease

The relationships between oral malodor and gingival or periodontal health are not as straightforward as in the case of the tongue. Conflicting data from various studies best demonstrate the complexity of this issue (Table 2.5).

Many earlier studies addressing this topic suggested a relationship between oral malodor and periodontal disease. Sulser and coworkers (Sulser et al. 1939) claimed that gingivitis and pyorrhea (i.e., periodontitis) are among the main conditions affecting breath odor concentration. Other researchers (Kostelc et al. 1984) found a significant increase in malodor-related compounds in experimental gingivitis.

Studies that compared malodor-related parameters in subjects with or without periodontal disease showed that oral sulfide levels were significantly higher in subjects with

Table 2.4 Correlations between tongue malodor scores and malodor-related parameters

References	Malodor-related parameters	Correlations
Kozlovsky et al. (1994) ($n = 52$)		*Pearson correlation*
	Tongue malodor[a] vs. oral malodor[b]	$r = 0.73$, $p < 0.001$
	Tongue malodor vs. sulfide monitor[c]	$r = 0.38$, $p = 0.003$
	Tongue malodor vs. pocket depth[d]	$r = 0.47$, $p = 0.005$
	Tongue malodor vs. GI[e]	$r = 0.47$, $p < 0.001$
	Tongue malodor vs. PI[f]	$r = 0.38$, $p = 0.003$
Bosy et al. (1994) ($n = 127$)		*Pearson correlation*
	Tongue malodor[a] vs. oral malodor[b]	$r = 0.55$, $p < 0.01$
	Tongue malodor vs. sulfide monitor[c]	$r = 0.40$, $p < 0.01$
	Tongue malodor vs. GI[e]	$r = 0.23$, $p < 0.01$
Greenstein et al. (1997) ($n = 123$)		*Pearson correlation*
	Tongue malodor[a] vs. oral malodor[b]	$r = 0.40$, $p < 0.001$
Sterer et al. (2002) ($n = 64$)		*Spearman correlation*
	Tongue malodor[a] vs. oral malodor[b]	
	Odor judge 1	$r = 0.63$, $p < 0.001$
	Odor judge 2	$r = 0.69$, $p < 0.001$
	Tongue malodor vs. sulfide monitor[c]	
	Odor judge 1	$r = 0.26$, $p = 0.036$
	Odor judge 2	$r = 0.38$, $p = 0.002$
Apatzidou et al. (2013) ($n = 78$)		*Spearman correlation*
	Tongue malodor[a] vs. oral malodor[b]	$r = 0.48$, $p < 0.001$
	Tongue malodor vs. sulfide monitor[c]	$r = 0.50$, $p < 0.001$

[a]Tongue coating malodor scored by an odor judge (0–5)
[b]Whole mouth malodor scored by an odor judge (0–5)
[c]Whole mouth ppb sulfide equivalents, Halimeter™
[d]Mean probing depth
[e]Gingival index (Löe and Silness 1963)
[f]Plaque index (Silness and Löe 1964)

Table 2.5 Oral malodor parameters and periodontal disease

References	Parameters/criteria	Findings
Kostelc et al. (1984) ($n = 10$)	Measurement of malodor-related compounds by gas chromatography in experimental gingivitis ($n = 5$) and controls ($n = 5$).	Significant increase in malodor related compounds in experimental gingivitis.
Rosenberg et al. (1991) ($n = 41$)		*Pearson correlation*
	Odor judge[a] 1 vs. pocket depth (no. >5 mm)	$r = 0.184$, $p = 0.047$
	Odor judge[a] 2 vs. pocket depth (no. >5 mm)	$r = 0.107$, NS[b]
	VSC[c] vs. pocket depth (no. >5 mm)	$r = 0.280$, $p = 0.002$
	Odor judge[a] 1 vs. gingival index[d]	$r = 0.099$, NS
	Odor judge[a] 2 vs. gingival index[d]	$r = 0.081$, NS
	VSC[c] vs. gingival index[d]	$r = 0.087$, $p = 0.053$
	Odor judge[a] 1 vs. plaque index[e]	$r = 0.353$, $p = 0.0001$
	Odor judge[a] 2 vs. plaque index[e]	$r = 0.359$, $p = 0.0001$
	VSC[c] vs. plaque index[e]	$r = 0.373$, $p = 0.0001$
	Odor judge[a] 1 vs. floss odor	$r = 0.381$, $p = 0.0001$
	Odor judge[a] 2 vs. floss odor	$r = 0.422$, $p = 0.0001$
	VSC[c] vs. floss odor	$r = 0.208$, $p = 0.026$
Yaegaki and Sanada (1992a) ($n = 31$)	Probing depth ≥ 4 mm is considered periodontal disease. Bleeding on probing (% BOP). VSC[f]	VSC is significantly higher in periodontal subjects. VSC is associated with bleeding on probing.
Bosy et al. (1994) ($n = 127$)		*Pearson correlation*
	Odor judge[a] vs. pocket depth (no. >5 mm)	$r = 0.11$, NS
	Odor judge[a] vs. gingival index[d]	$r = 0.15$, NS
	Odor judge[a] vs. plaque index[e]	$r = 0.12$, NS
	Odor judge[a] vs. floss odor	$r = 0.23$, $p < 0.01$

Table 2.5   (continued)

References	Parameters/criteria		Findings
De Boever et al. (1994) ($n = 55$)	Malodor complaint	No complaint	Differences between groups (ANOVA)
	Odor judge[g]		$P < 0.005$
	VSC[h]		$P < 0.05$
	Bleeding on probing (% BOP)		$P < 0.005$
Kozlovsky et al. (1994) ($n = 52$)			*Pearson correlation*
	Odor judge[a] vs. mean pocket depth		$r = 0.581$, $p < 0.001$
	VSC[c] vs. mean pocket depth		$r = 0.305$, $p = 0.050$
	Odor judge[a] vs. gingival index[d]		$r = 0.536$, $p < 0.001$
	VSC[c] vs. gingival index[d]		$r = 0.298$, $p = 0.017$
	Odor judge[a] vs. plaque index[e]		$r = 0.383$, $p = 0.003$
	VSC[c] vs. plaque index[e]		$r = 0.188$, $p = 0.093$
Soder et al. (2000) ($n = 1681$)	Foetor ex ore (severe malodor) Probing depth scores (% of teeth with probing depth >5 mm). Gingival index scores (redness swelling and bleeding)		Subject with severe malodor ($n = 41$) had significantly higher probing depth and gingival index scores ($p < 0.001$)
Morita and Wang (2001) ($n = 81$)			*Pearson correlation*
	Odor judge[a] vs. pocket depth (%≥6 mm)		$r = 0.371$, $p = 0.001$
	VSC[h] vs. pocket depth (% ≥ 6 mm)		$r = 0.411$, $p < 0.001$
	Odor judge[a] vs. bleeding on probing (%)		$r = 0.489$, $p < 0.001$
	VSC[h] vs. bleeding on probing (%)		$r = 0.472$, $p < 0.001$
Figueiredo et al. (2002)	Probing >3 mm ($n = 21$)	Probing ≤3 mm ($n = 20$)	Differences between groups (ANOVA)
	Odor judge[g]		$p = 0.001$
	VSC[h]		$p = 0.02$
	Gingival index[c]		$p = 0.005$
	Plaque index[e]		$p = 0.006$
Stamou et al. (2005) ($n = 71$)			*Pearson correlation*
	Odor judge[a] vs. probing depth		$r = -0.054$, NS
	Odor judge[a] vs. gingival index[d]		$r = 0.185$, NS
	Odor judge[a] vs. plaque index[e]		$r = 0.111$, NS

Table 2.5   (continued)

References	Parameters/criteria	Findings
Tsai et al. (2008) ($n = 72$)		*Pearson correlation*
	Odor judge[a] vs. pocket depth (%>5 mm)	$r = 0.22$, NS
	Odor judge[a] vs. bleeding on probing (%)	$r = 0.54$, $p < 0.001$
Bolepalli et al. (2015) ($n = 240$)		*Pearson correlation*
	Odor judge[a] vs. mean pocket depth	$r = 0.726$, $p < 0.001$
	VSC[h] vs. mean pocket depth	$r = 0.662$, $p < 0.001$
	Odor judge[a] vs. bleeding on probing (%)	$r = 0.908$, $p < 0.001$
	VSC[h] vs. bleeding on probing (%)	$r = 0.816$, $p < 0.001$
	Odor judge[a] vs. gingival index[d]	$r = 0.844$, $p < 0.001$
	VSC[h] vs. gingival index[d]	$r = 0.747$, $p < 0.001$
	Odor judge[a] vs. plaque index[e]	$r = 0.836$, $p < 0.001$
	VSC[h] vs. plaque index[e]	$r = 0.722$, $p < 0.001$

[a]Odor judge scores on a scale of 0–5
[b]NS—nonsignificant
[c]Volatile sulfide compounds measured by sulfide monitor (1170)
[d]Gingival index (GI; Löe and Silness 1963)
[e]Plaque index (PI; Silness and Löe 1964)
[f]Volatile sulfide compounds (VSC) measured by gas chromatography
[g]Odor judge scores on a scale of 0–4
[h]Volatile sulfide compounds measured by Halimeter

periodontal pocket depths of 4 mm or more (Yaegaki and Sanada 1992a, b), and that subjects with periodontal disease (pocket depth > 3 mm) had significantly higher malodor ratings as scored by an odor judge (Figueiredo et al. 2002). In another study (Soder et al. 2000), subjects with severe oral malodor (*Foetor ex ore*) had a significantly higher percentage of teeth with periodontal pocket depths of at least 5 mm as well as higher gingival index scores (redness, swelling, and bleeding). Furthermore, large studies done in Japan (Miyazaki et al. 1995), China (Liu et al. 2006), and Switzerland (Bornstein et al. 2009) also found significant correlations comparing oral malodor and periodontal status (Table 2.2).

In contrast, a study by Bosy and coworkers (Bosy et al. 1994) found no association between oral malodor and periodontal disease (pocket depth ≥ 5 mm), suggesting that these may be two independent conditions. Another more recent study by Tsai and coworkers (2008) also failed to show an association between malodor levels and the percentage of teeth with periodontal involvement (pocket depth ≥ 5 mm). However, the latter did find an association between malodor levels and the percentage of teeth with bleeding on probing.

To further complicate matters, some studies (Yaegaki and Sanada 1992a, b) reported that subjects with periodontal disease (probing depth ≥ 4 mm) had significantly more tongue coating (four times more wet weight) than the control non-periodontal subjects. These studies further showed that the tongue coating was responsible for production of 60% of the malodor-related volatile sulfide compounds and that these compounds were associated with the percentage of sites exhibiting bleeding on probing.

These data, taken together, suggest that regarding malodor production, periodontal disease is less dominant than tongue coating. It is also apparent that the active inflammation process is the main link between gingival and periodontal disease and malodor production, rather than past evidence of periodontal disease. Active gingivitis (Fig. 2.2) or periodontitis, represented

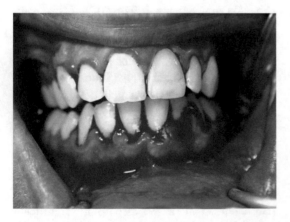

Fig. 2.2 Gingivitis; swollen bleading gums showing signs of inflammation (kindly provided by Dr. M. Perez-Davidi)

by one of its chief signs (i.e., bleeding on probing or papillary bleeding), accompanied by bacterial activity, increased flow of crevicular fluid, and presence of blood cells seems more relevant to the malodor production process than the presence or depth of periodontal pockets. The inflammatory process may be further exacerbated by the malodorous compounds, which are for the most part toxic and increase tissue permeability and damage (Ng and Tonzetich 1984).

2.3   Oral Malodor and Dental Restorations

As a rule, any appliance, fixed or removable, within the oral cavity which hinders the common practice of oral hygiene and facilitates plaque accumulation, has the potential to increase oral malodor production.

Dental crowns and bridges are the most common examples of this principle. Dental bridges in particular form an obstacle to maintaining good interdental hygiene by preventing regular flossing. This is also true for orthodontic appliances and splints. Studies conducted on oral malodor in patients with fixed orthodontic appliances showed significant increase in malodor levels as early as 1 week following bonding (Babacan et al. 2011; Nalçacı et al. 2014) concomitantly with rises in plaque scores and gingival inflammation.

In addition, faulty restorations, particularly if ill fitted or decemented, may even intensify the problem by allowing bacterial proliferation and accumulation in the inner gaps between the prepared tooth and the restoration, thus forming a reservoir of anaerobic bacteria.

Another such reservoir has been demonstrated in the inner space of the implant–abutment interface (IAI) of osseointegrated dental implants. Research showed that when this interface is situated over 2 mm in depth with respect to the surrounding soft tissue, the inner compartment of the implant harbors significantly more malodor-producing bacteria as compared to implants with shallower transmucosal depth (Sterer et al. 2008).

Acrylic appliances such as dentures and obturators are known for their plaque-accumulating properties. Their porotic nature and increased tendency to adsorb salivary proteins, resulting in bacterial adhesion, turn the acrylic appliance into a bacterial reservoir. Although little research has been carried out on the composition of denture biofilm, in a study performed by Goldberg and coworkers (Goldberg et al. 1997), certain types of malodor-producing bacteria, not normally considered important members of the oral microbiota (i.e., Enterobacteriaceae), were shown to be dramatically increased in the case of dentures wearers. Furthermore, when cultivated in the lab, these bacteria produce malodor similar to denture malodor.

Apart from bacterial accumulation and denture contamination, it seems that behavioral aspects also play a part in denture-related malodor. Research done on denture wearing habits and malodor showed that malodor-related compounds were significantly increased in subjects who did not remove their dentures during the night (Nalcaci and Baran 2008).

2.4 Oral Malodor and Oral Dryness

Saliva has an important role in maintaining oral health and many oral functions (e.g., eating, talking). However, being comprised of 98% water, it also provides suitable moist environment leading to an abundance of microorganisms within the oral cavity.

These bacteria produce many metabolic byproducts and waste materials as a result of their activity, many of which (described further in Chap. 3) are foul smelling. Some of these bacterial byproducts are more volatile than others. However, when there is a decrease in saliva flow and the oral mucosa becomes dry some of the less volatile compounds may escape the oral surfaces, and become detected on the breath. These and other possible mechanisms (e.g., lack of salivary antibacterial and washing effect, as well as salivary stagnation and degradation of salivary glycoproteins) may explain why decreasing saliva flow increases the severity of malodor in individual subjects. In studies comparing saliva flow and malodor-related compounds (Koshimune et al. 2003; Suzuki et al. 2016), lower levels of resting saliva flow (e.g., without stimulating saliva flow by chewing) were associated with higher levels of malodor-related compounds and high malodor ratings (odor judge scores $\geq$3).

There are several physiological conditions that affect saliva flow. For example, during sleep saliva flow is brought to a halt (Dawes 1972). That is one of the reasons that sleep, especially when accompanied by mouth breathing, may promote oral malodor production. In addition, mouth breathing on its own has been shown to be associated with increased levels of oral malodor (Motta et al. 2011). Normally, saliva flow decreases between meals. Dehydration due to insufficient fluid intake and prolonged fasting may also result in reduced saliva flow.

Another condition that might affect saliva flow is stress. Research by Quciroz and coworkers (Queiroz et al. 2002) showed that stress can cause salivary flow reduction and concomitant increase in malodor-related compounds. Anxiety was also shown to elevate these compounds (Calil and Marcondes 2006). However, other researchers showed that stress-induced elevation in VSC production was not associated with saliva flow, but was affected by gender (Lima et al. 2013).

Many widely used medications such as antihypertensive and antidepressants drugs are known to have reducing effect on saliva flow as an undesirable side effect. The use of such drugs, as well as increased consumption of coffee and alcohol, may cause an increase in malodor production as a result of salivary flow decrease (Tschoppe et al. 2010).

Unlike conditions that cause a temporary reduction in resting saliva flow, chronic dry mouth conditions (i.e., xerostomia) which are often accompanied by a subjective complaint of halitosis do not seem to increase malodor levels. In a recent study conducted on 58 primary Sjögren's syndrome patients, 22 non-Sjögren's syndrome sicca patients and 57 age matching healthy control subjects, no difference was observed between the groups in malodor and VSC levels (Singh et al. 2019). One possible explanation for this might be the low pH conditions usually associated with xerostomia that may hinder malodor production (for more details, see Chap. 2).

References

Amou T, Hinode D, Yoshioka M, Grenier D. Relationship between halitosis and periodontal disease—associated oral bacteria in tongue coatings. Int J Dent Hyg. 2014;12(2):145–51.

Apatzidou AD, Bakirtzoglou E, Vouros I, Karagiannis V, Papa A, Konstantinidis A. Association between oral malodour and periodontal disease-related parameters in the general population. Acta Odontol Scand. 2013;71(1):189–95.

Avincsal MO, Altundag A, Dinc ME, Cayonu M, Topak M, Kulekci M. Evaluation of halitosis using OralChroma™ in patients with allergic rhinitis. Eur Ann Otorhinolaryngol Head Neck Dis. 2016;133(4):243–6.

Babacan H, Sokucu O, Marakoglu I, Ozdemir H, Nalcaci R. Effect of fixed appliances on oral malodor. Am J Orthod Dentofacial Orthop. 2011;139(3):351–5.

Bolepalli AC, Munireddy C, Peruka S, Polepalle T, Choudary Alluri LS, Mishaeel S. Determining the association between oral malodor and periodontal disease: a case control study. J Int Soc Prev Community Dent. 2015;5(5):413–8.

Bornstein MM, Kislig K, Hoti BB, Seemann R, Lussi A. Prevalence of halitosis in the population of the city of Bern, Switzerland: a study comparing self-reported and clinical data. Eur J Oral Sci. 2009;117(3):261–7.

Bosy A, Kulkarni GV, Rosenberg M, McCulloch CA. Relationship of oral malodor to periodontitis: evidence of independence in discrete subpopulations. J Periodontol. 1994;65(1):37–46.

Bretz WA, Biesbrock A, Corby PM, Corby AL, Bretz WG, Wessel J, Schork NJ. Environmental and genetic contributions to indicators of oral malodor in twins. Twin Res Hum Genet. 2011;14(6):568–72.

Calil CM, Marcondes FK. Influence of anxiety on the production of oral volatile sulfur compounds. Life Sci. 2006;79(7):660–4.

Dawes C. Circadian rhythms in human salivary flow rate and composition. J Physiol. 1972;220(3):529–45.

De Boever EH, De Uzeda M, Loesche WJ. Relationship between volatile sulfur compounds, BANA-hydrolyzing bacteria and gingival health in patients with and without complaints of oral malodor. J Clin Dent. 1994;4(4):114–9.

Delanghe G, Ghyselen J, Feenstra L, Van Steenberghe D. Experiences of a Belgian multidisciplinary breath odour clinic. In: Van Steenberghe D, Rosenberg M, editors. Bad breath a multy disciplinary approach. Leuven: Leuven University Press; 1996. p. 199–208.

Figueiredo LC, Rosetti EP, Marcantonio E Jr, Marcantonio RA, Salvador SL. The relationship of oral malodor in patients with or without periodontal disease. J Periodontol. 2002;73(11):1338–42.

Goldberg S, Cardash H, Browning H 3rd, Sahly H, Rosenberg M. Isolation of Enterobacteriaceae from the mouth and potential association with malodor. J Dent Res. 1997;76(11):1770–5.

Grapp GL. Fetor oris (halitosis): a medical and dental responsibility. Northwest Med. 1933;32:375–80.

Greenstein RB, Goldberg S, Marku-Cohen S, Sterer N, Rosenberg M. Reduction of oral malodor by oxidizing lozenges. J Periodontol. 1997;68(12):1176–81.

Gross A, Barnes GP, Lyon TC. Effects of tongue brushing on tongue coating and dental plaque scores. J Dent Res. 1975;54(6):1236.

Haraszthy VI, Zambon JJ, Sreenivasan PK, Zambon MM, Gerber D, Rego R, Parker C. Identification of oral bacterial species associated with halitosis. J Am Dent Assoc. 2007;138(8):1113–20.

Kim J, Jung Y, Park K, Park JW. A digital tongue imaging system for tongue coating evaluation in patients with oral malodour. Oral Dis. 2009;15(8):565–9.

Koshimune S, Awano S, Gohara K, Kurihara E, Ansai T, Takehara T. Low salivary flow and volatile sulfur compounds in mouth air. Oral Surg Oral Med Oral Pathol Oral Radiol Endod. 2003;96(1):38–41.

Kostelc JG, Preti G, Zelson PR, Brauner L, Baehni P. Oral odors in early experimental gingivitis. J Periodontal Res. 1984;19(3):303–12.

Kozlovsky A, Gordon D, Gelernter I, Loesche WJ, Rosenberg M. Correlation between the BANA test and oral malodor parameters. J Dent Res. 1994;73(5):1036–42.

Lee ES, Yim HK, Lee HS, Choi JH, Lee JH, Kim BI. Clinical assessment of oral malodor using autofluorescence of tongue coating. Photodiagnosis Photodyn Ther. 2016;13:323–9.

Lima PO, Calil CM, Marcondes FK. Influence of gender and stress on the volatile sulfur compounds and stress biomarkers production. Oral Dis. 2013;19(4):366–73.

Liu XN, Shinada K, Chen XC, Zhang BX, Yaegaki K, Kawaguchi Y. Oral malodor-related parameters in the Chinese general population. J Clin Periodontol. 2006;33(1):31–6.

Löe H, Silness J. Periodontal disease in pregnancy. I Prevalence and Severity. Acta Odontol Scand. 1963;21:533–51.

Mantilla Gomez S, Danser MM, Sipos PM, Rowshani B, van der Velden U, van der Weijden GA. Tongue coating and salivary bacterial counts in healthy/gingivitis subjects and periodontitis patients. J Clin Periodontol. 2001;28(10):970–8.

Miyazaki H, Sakao S, Katoh Y, Takehara T. Correlation between volatile sulphur compounds and certain oral health measurements in the general population. J Periodontol. 1995;66(8):679–84.

Morita M, Wang HL. Relationship between sulcular sulfide level and oral malodor in subjects with periodontal disease. J Periodontol. 2001;72(1):79–84.

Morita M, Musinski DL, Wang HL. Assessment of newly developed tongue sulfide probe for detecting oral malodor. J Clin Periodontol. 2001;28(5):494–6.

Motta LJ, Bachiega JC, Guedes CC, Laranja LT, Bussadori SK. Association between halitosis and mouth breathing in children. Clinics (Sao Paulo). 2011;66(6):939–42.

Nalcaci R, Baran I. Oral malodor and removable complete dentures in the elderly. Oral Surg Oral Med Oral Pathol Oral Radiol Endod. 2008;105(6):e5–9.

Nalçacı R, Özat Y, Çokakoğlu S, Türkkahraman H, Önal S, Kaya S. Effect of bracket type on halitosis, periodontal status, and microbial colonization. Angle Orthod. 2014;84(3):479–85.

Ng W, Tonzetich J. Effect of hydrogen sulfide and methyl mercaptan on the permeability of oral mucosa. J Dent Res. 1984;63(7):994–7.

Oho T, Yoshida Y, Shimazaki Y, Yamashita Y, Koga T. Characteristics of patients complaining of halitosis and the usefulness of gas chromatography for diagnosing halitosis. Oral Surg Oral Med Oral Pathol Oral Radiol Endod. 2001;91(5):531–4.

Queiroz CS, Hayacibara MF, Tabchoury CP, Marcondes FK, Cury JA. Relationship between stressful situations, salivary flow rate and oral volatile sulfur-containing compounds. Eur J Oral Sci. 2002;110(5):337–40.

Quirynen M, Dadamio J, Van den Velde S, De Smit M, Dekeyser C, Van Tornout M, Vandekerckhove B. Characteristics of 2000 patients who visited a halitosis clinic. J Clin Periodontol. 2009;36(11):970–5.

Rosenberg M. Clinical assessment of bad breath: current concepts. J Am Dent Assoc. 1996;127(4):475–82.

Rosenberg M, Kulkarni GV, Bosy A, McCulloch CA. Reproducibility and sensitivity of oral malodor measurements with a portable sulphide monitor. J Dent Res. 1991;70(11):1436–40.

Seemann R, Bizhang M, Djamchidi C, Kage A, Nachnani S. The proportion of pseudo-halitosis patients in a multidisciplinary breath malodour consultation. Int Dent J. 2006;56(2):77–81.

Silness J, Löe H. Periodontal disease in pregnancy. II. Correlation between oral hygiene and periodontal condition. Acta Odontol Scand. 1964;22:121–35.

Singh PB, Young A, Homayouni A, Hove LH, Petrovski BÉ, Herlofson BB, Palm Ø, Rykke M, Jensen JL. Distorted taste and impaired oral health in patients with sicca complaints. Nutrients. 2019;11(2):E264.

Soder B, Johansson B, Soder PO. The relation between foetor ex ore, oral hygiene and periodontal disease. Swed Dent J. 2000;24(3):73–82.

Stamou E, Kozlovsky A, Rosenberg M. Association between oral malodour and periodontal disease-related parameters in a population of 71 Israelis. Oral Dis. 2005;11(Suppl 1):72–4.

Sterer N, Greenstein RB, Rosenberg M. Beta-galactosidase activity in saliva is associated with oral malodor. J Dent Res. 2002;81(3):182–5.

Sterer N, Tamary I, Katz M, Weiss E. Association between transmucosal depth of osseointegrated implants and malodor production. Int J Oral Maxillofac Implants. 2008;23(2):277–80.

Sulser GF, Brening RH, Fosdick LS. Some conditions that effect the odor concentration of breath. J Dent Res. 1939;18(4):355–9.

Suzuki N, Fujimoto A, Yoneda M, Watanabe T, Hirofuji T, Hanioka T. Resting salivary flow independently associated with oral malodor. BMC Oral Health. 2016;17(1):23.

Tonzetich J, Ng SK. Reduction of malodor by oral cleansing procedures. Oral Surg Oral Med Oral Pathol. 1976;42(2):172–81.

Tsai CC, Chou HH, Wu TL, Yang YH, Ho KY, Wu YM, Ho YP. The levels of volatile sulfur compounds in mouth air from patients with chronic periodontitis. J Periodontal Res. 2008;43(2):186–93.

Tschoppe P, Wolgin M, Pischon N, Kielbassa AM. Etiologic factors of hyposalivation and consequences for oral health. Quintessence Int. 2010;41(4):321–33.

Washio J, Sato T, Koseki T, Takahashi N. Hydrogen sulfide-producing bacteria in tongue biofilm and their relationship with oral malodour. J Med Microbiol. 2005;54(Pt 9):889–95.

Winkel EG, Roldan S, Van Winkelhoff AJ, Herrera D, Sanz M. Clinical effects of a new mouthrinse containing chlorhexidine, cetylpyridinium chloride and zinc-lactate on oral halitosis. A dual-center, double-blind placebo-controlled study. J Clin Periodontol. 2003;30(4):300–6.

Yaegaki K, Sanada K. Volatile sulfur compounds in mouth air from clinically healthy subjects and patients with periodontal disease. J Periodontal Res. 1992a;27(4 Pt 1):233–8.

Yaegaki K, Sanada K. Biochemical and clinical factors influencing oral malodor in periodontal patients. J Periodontol. 1992b;63(9):783–9.

Zürcher A, Filippi A. Findings, diagnoses and results of a halitosis clinic over a seven year period. Schweiz Monatsschr Zahnmed. 2012;122(3):205–16.

Biochemical and Microbial Aspects of Oral Malodor Production

3

Contents

3.1 The General Role of Bacteria in Breath Odors

There is ample evidence that in the large majority of cases, oral malodor derives from bacterial activity within the oral cavity. It is also likely that most cases of odor deriving from the nasal passages and tonsils are also bacterial in origin. One indication for this is the transient reduction of oral malodor observed following local antiseptic treatment (e.g., mouthwash), and the elimination of almost all cases of halitosis following systemic antibiotic treatment.

In a larger context, bacteria are responsible for many of the foul odors that we encounter in everyday lives (e.g., sewage, animal waste, garbage and spoiled food, contaminated water, body odor, etc.)

Bacteria produce a wide variety of foul odors depending on the substrates being degraded, and the metabolic pathways involved. It is possible that through our evolution we have learned to detest these types of odor components as a health hazard warning.

In the oral cavity itself hundreds of species cohabit the many available niches, living in different microenvironments and feeding on a variety of organic substrates. It is here that most cases of bad breath begin.

3.2 The Bacterial Origin of Oral Odors

The diverse microbial population of the oral cavity can be divided according to various metabolic characteristics such as nutritional requirements and oxygen tolerance. The Gram-positive oral bacteria are generally saccharolytic and facultative in nature, i.e., that they degrade and utilize

© Springer Nature Switzerland AG 2020
N. Sterer, M. Rosenberg, *Breath Odors*, https://doi.org/10.1007/978-3-030-44731-1_3

monosaccharides, disaccharides, and carbohydrates as their main energy source (e.g., fermentation) and can consume oxygen in the process. Members of this group such as Streptococci and Actinomyces spp. are often considered to be early colonizers of the oral biofilm, and some Gram-positive (e.g. mutans streptococci) are blamed for fermenting sugars into acids and causing dental caries.

The Gram-negative oral bacteria on the other hand are generally considered to be proteolytic and anaerobic. These types of bacteria often prefer anaerobic conditions (i.e., lack of oxygen) for growth and utilize proteins, peptides, and amino acids as a major source of carbon, nitrogen, and energy (i.e., putrefaction). Some members of the Gram-negative community (e.g., *Fusobacterium, Treponema, Porphyromonas,* and *Prevotella*) are considered to be particularly implicated in periodontal diseases and malodor production.

To avoid being swallowed or washed away, oral bacteria adhere to surfaces as well as to each other, forming multilayer microscopic structures known as oral biofilms. The bacteria dominating the outer exposed layers of the oral biofilms throughout the mouth are either aerobic or aerotolerant, surviving under relatively high oxidation (E_h) levels. Following maturation and succession of these microniches, oxygen depletion by microbes in the outer levels allows for the proliferation of increasingly anaerobic species. In the laboratory, Gram-positive microorganisms are generally found to inhabit the outer layers of oral biofilms, and Gram-negative anaerobes thrive in the reduced inner layers.

3.3   Metabolic Factors Affecting Malodor Production

pH and Glucose Fosdick and colleagues (Berg et al. 1946) reported that the putrefaction rate of incubated saliva samples is strongly inhibited in the presence of even a small amount of sugar, but gave no possible explanation for this observation.

In 1972, McNamara and coworkers (1972) reported that whole saliva, adjusted to slightly acidic conditions (pH 6.5) did not produce malodor following incubation, whereas at pH 7.5 malodor was produced. This study also showed that the addition of glucose to incubated saliva prevents malodor production and causes an increase in the proportion of Gram-positive bacteria. McNamara concluded that glucose fermentation and resulting acidity inactivated amino acid metabolism and favored the growth of saccharolytic Gram-positive bacteria.

Kleinberg and Codipilly (1997) also demonstrated, using a salivary incubation assay, that the addition of glucose results in pH reduction and concomitant inhibition of malodor production. They concluded that acidic pH is inhibitory to bacterial metabolism leading to malodor formation. Whereas, the saccharolytic Gram-positive oral bacteria reduce the pH by fermentation and acid production (e.g., lactic acid), the proteolytic Gram-negative oral bacteria tend to increase the pH by putrefaction (e.g., urea production). Furthermore, the activity of the various enzymes involved (e.g., saccharolytic, proteolytic) is optimal in different pH ranges.

Another possible explanation for the effect of acidity on malodor inhibition was proposed by Tonzetich and coworkers (1967). They suggested that various pH conditions may affect the volatility traits of the malodor components.

Oxygen Depletion and Redox Potential Oxygen depletion and reduced E_h are imperative for the development of malodor-producing anaerobic Gram-negative oral bacteria.

Berg and Fosdick (1946) showed that anaerobic conditions increased salivary putrefaction and malodor production. Kleinberg (Codipilly et al. 2004) showed that low E_h readings highly correlated with oral malodor ratings. Greenstein and colleagues (1997) demonstrated that the rate of oxygen depletion by saliva samples from human subjects correlated with oral malodor-related parameters. Furthermore, we have recently shown that volatile sulfide compounds are produced in the deep layers of mature oral biofilm where anaerobic conditions predominate (Sterer et al. 2009; Fig. 3.1).

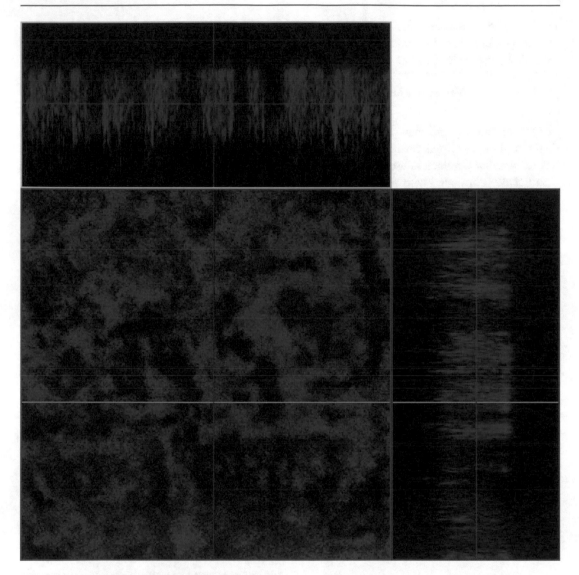

Fig. 3.1 VSC production in biofilm

3.4 Biochemical Aspects

3.4.1 Metabolism

Oral malodor is considered to derive primarily from the anaerobic degradation of protein-aceous materials by oral microorganisms. Proteins are readily available from saliva, exfoliated epithelial cells, food debris, blood, and crevicular fluids and possibly postnasal drip. The constituent proteins are hydrolyzed by proteolytic enzymes of bacterial origin, yielding free amino acids which can then be further broken down. Some of the molecular by-products of this process are particularly foul-smelling.

Protein → Amino acids → Putrefactive end products

(source: Fosdick and Piez 1953)

Deglycosylation Salivary mucins are large glyco-proteins comprised of a long protein core surrounded by carbohydrate side chains in a bottle brush-like structure. Unlike ordinary polypeptides, their proteolytic degradation requires the prior removal of their carbohydrate side chains, or deglycosylation.

$$\text{Mucin} \rightarrow \text{Protein} \rightarrow \text{Amino acids} \rightarrow \text{Putrefactive end products}$$

One of the key enzymes in salivary mucin deglycosylation is β-galactosidase. Our research has shown that β-galactosidase activity in saliva significantly correlated with malodor ratings of 64 subjects (Sterer et al. 2002). Furthermore, addition of β-galactosidase or β-galactosidase-producing bacteria (i.e., *Streptococcus salivarius*) to a mucin incubation mixture promoted mucin putrefaction by *Porphyromonas gingivalis* (Sterer and Rosenberg 2006).

The proteolytic process described above results in the breakdown of available oral proteins (or glycoproteins) into free amino acids. These free amino acids serve as nutrients for oral microorganisms that do not grow on carbohydrates (asacharolytic), and their metabolites are important pH modulators and precursors for various molecules such as iron-scavenging sidero-phores. Amino acids are degraded via different metabolic pathways such as deamination (Table 3.1), decarboxylation (Table 3.2), and various oxidation–reduction processes, yielding different by-products, as described below.

Volatile Fatty Acids The enzymatic cleavage of the amino group from various amino acids occurs at a pH range of 6–7 and results in the production of volatile fatty acids and ammonia (NH_3).

$$\overset{\displaystyle NH_2}{\underset{\displaystyle |}{P\text{–}XH}} - XOOH + H_2O \rightarrow R\text{ - }COOH + NH_3 + 4H + CO_2$$

Amines Decarboxylation of nitrogen containing amino acids occurs in the mouth mainly at pH 6.5 (Gochman et al. 1959) and serves also as a means for the microorganisms to regulate pH conditions. The decarboxylation of these amino acids results in the production of various amine compounds.

$$\overset{\displaystyle NH_2}{\underset{\displaystyle |}{R\text{-}CH}} - COOH \rightarrow R\text{ - }CH_2 - NH_2 + CO_2 + H$$

Table 3.1 Deamination products of anaerobic bacteria

Amino acid	VFA produced
Alanine, glycine, serine	Acetate
Threonine	Propionate
Glutamate, aspartate	Acetate, propionate, butyrate
Valine	Isobutyrate
Leucine	Isovalerate
Isoleucine	2-methylbutyrate
Phenylalanine	Phenylacetate
Tyrosine	*p*-Hydroxyphenylacetate
Tryptophan	Indoleacetate → 3-methylindole
Tyrosine	Phenylacetate, phenylpropionate

Source: Mackie et al. (1998)

Table 3.2 Decarboxylation reactions by anaerobic bacteria

Amino acid	Amine produced
Glycine	Methylamine
Alanine	Ethylamine
α-Aminobutyrate	Propylamine
Ornithine	Putrescine → pyrrolidine[a]
Arginine[b]	Putrescine → pyrrolidine[a]
Norvaline	Butylamine
Lysine	Cadaverine → piperidine[a]
Arginine	Agmatine
Histidine	Histamine
Cysteic acid	Taurine
Tyrosine	Tyramine
Tryptophan	Tryptamine
Phenylalanine	Phenylethylamine

Source: Mackie et al. (1998)
[a]Ring closure reaction
[b]Decarboxylation and hydrolysis

Table 3.3 Indoles and phenols

Amino acid	Products
Tyrosine	Phenol, p-Cresol
Tryptophan	Indole, 3-methylindole (Skatole)
Phenylalanine	Phenyl acetate, phenylpropionate

Source: Mackie et al. (1998)

Indoles and Phenols Production of indoles and phenols occurs as a result of the metabolism of various aromatic amino acids (Table 3.3).

Volatile Sulfide Compounds Production of sulfur-containing compounds results from sulfate reduction or the metabolism of sulfur-containing amino acids

$$Cysteine \rightarrow Hydrogen\ sulfide$$

$$Methionine \rightarrow Methyl\ mercaptan$$

3.4.2 Malodorous Volatile Organic Compounds (VOCs) in the Oral Cavity

Many of the above compounds, as well as various other volatile organic compounds (VOCs), have been detected in saliva samples, saliva headspace, tongue coating samples, and breath samples (Table 3.4). These samples were analyzed using different techniques varying from classic colorimetric techniques to modern liquid and gas chromatography. These reported compounds are listed below, highlighting those that have been implicated in oral malodor production and stating their odor characteristics and thresholds:

Research on malodorous volatile organic compounds (VOCs) from the oral cavity was initially carried out using salivary putrefaction assays. Whole saliva was stimulated by chewing on paraffin wax and incubated under various conditions (e.g., aerobic, anaerobic) with or without adding additional nutrients or inhibitors (e.g., amino acids, glucose). Early work done by Fosdick and colleagues in the 1940s and 1950s on salivary putrefaction and periodontal disease showed that amines, indoles, and sulfides are produced in putrefied saliva concomitant with malodor production especially if the saliva is incubated anaerobically in the presence of additional protein (Berg et al. 1946; Fosdick and Piez 1953).

Studies done by Tonzetich and Richter (1964) during the 1960s using saliva from healthy subjects, demonstrated the importance of volatile sulfide compounds (VSCs, especially hydrogen sulfide and methyl mercaptan) as major detectable components of oral malodor. According to Tonzetich, volatile sulfides are the only compounds that play a meaningful part in odor production. He showed that adding sulfur-containing amino acid such as cysteine to the incubation mixture (precursor of hydrogen sulfide) caused increased malodor production, whereas the addition of nitrogen-containing amino acid such as arginine (precursor of putrescine) or aromatic amino acid such as tryptophan (precursor of indole) did not. Tonzetich claimed that the reason for the inability of amines and indoles, despite their foul smell and low odor threshold, to increase salivary malodor, was their low volatility (Tonzetich et al. 1967).

During the early 1970s, Tonzetich and colleagues reported the use of gas chromatography coupled to a flame-photometric detector for the chemical analysis of breath malodor (Tonzetich 1971). Their findings linking volatile sulfides and malodor seemed to confirm the hegemony of volatile sulfide compounds as the major malodorous components of breath malodor.

This viewpoint, however, has been challenged by other researchers, especially Kleinberg and colleagues. They demonstrated that oral dryness can increase the concentration of volatiles (Kleinberg et al. 2002). Furthermore, they showed that when the aqueous solutions of odoriferous volatiles are allowed to dry on the skin, the smells of some amines, indoles, and volatile fatty acids (VFA) are more pronounced and linger much longer then the smell of the volatile sulfides (Kleinberg and Codipilly 1997). Kleinberg also showed that incubating pure cultures of Gram-negative oral bacteria in the presence of various amino acids, including nitrogen containing and aromatic, did result in malodor production. Other researchers have also demonstrated

Table 3.4 Oral VOCs detected in saliva, tongue coating samples, saliva headspace, and mouth air

Compound	Odor description	Odor threshold (ppm v/v)	Refs
Acids			
Acetic acid			(2, 6)
Butyric acid			(2, 6)
Methylpropionic acid			(2)
Methylpropanoic acid			(10)
Alcohols			
Ethanol			(1)
Propanol			(1, 4, 5, 6, 10)
Hexanol			(10)
Decanol			(1)
Butanol			(10)
Dodecanol			(1)
Tetradecanol			(1)
Hexadecanol			(1)
Phenylethanol			(1)
2-ethylhexanol			(1)
Benzylalcohol			(1)
Aldehydes			
2-heptanal			(2)
2-octanal			(2)
Nonanal			(5, 10)
Decanal			(10)
Propanal			(10)
Acetaldehyde			(6)
Benzaldehyde			(1, 5)
Aromatics			
C_2–C_4 alkyl benzenes			(1, 10)
Ethylbenzene			(2)
Styrene			(1, 5)
Dimethylbenzene			(2)
Benzene			(1, 10)
Cadalene			(10)
Naphtalene			(2)
Toluene			(1, 10)
Ethers			
Dimethylfuran			(1, 10)
Butylfuran			(10)
Anethole			(10)
Estragole			(10)
Fixed gases			
Carbon disulfide			(4)
Dimethyl selenide			(4)
Thiopropanal-*S*-oxide			(6)
Hydrocarbons			
2-Methyl-propane			(2)
Dimethoxy-methane			(2)
Trichloro-ethane			(2)
1(1 ethoxyethoxy)-propane			(2)
2-methyl 1-nitropropane			(2)
2,4-pentadienenitryl			(2)
Isoprene			(5)

Table 3.4 (continued)

Compound	Odor description	Odor threshold (ppm v/v)	Refs
Caryophyllene			(5)
β-Pinene			(5)
Isobutene			**(5)**
Tridecane			(5)
Dodecane			(5, 10)
Heptane			(10)
Hexane			(10)
Nonane			(10)
Undecane			(5, 10)
Pentadecane			(5)
Decane			(5)
Limonene			(2, 5, 10)
C_8–C_{12} alkanes			(1)
C_{17} alkane			(1)
Ketones			
2-butanone			(4, 5, 10)
2-decanone			(10)
2-nonanone			(10)
2-octanone			(10)
2-heptanone			(2)
2-hexanone			(2)
2-pentanone			(4)
6-methyl-2-heptanone			(2)
Acetone			(1, 4, 5, 6, 10)
Nitrogen-containing compounds			
Diphenylamine			(1)
Pyrrolidine			(2, 10)
Putrescine			(3, 7)
Cadaverine	Putrid	–	(3, **7**)
Methenamine	–	–	**(5)**
Ammonia	Pungent	1.5	(6, **8**)
Indole	Fecal	0.00030	(1, 2, 3, 4, **9**, 10)
2-methyl pyridine (Picoline)	Sweat	0.031	(**1**, 2)
3-methyl pyridine			**(1)**
4-methyl pyridine			**(1)**
Ethyl-pyridine			(2)
3-methyl-indole (Skatole)	Fecal	0.0000056	(1, 2, 3, 4, 10)
Pyridine	Rancid	0.063	**(1)**
Acetonitrile			(10)
Thiazole			(10)
Phenols			
p-Cresol			(1, 2)
Dimethylphenol			(2)
Phenol			(1, 2, 5)
Sulfur-containing compounds			
2-methyl-thio-propane			(2)
Mercaptoacetic acid (2)			(2)
Methylsufhide (2)			(2)
Propane–thiol (2)			(2)
Methylthiopropane (2)			(2, 10)

(continued)

Table 3.4 (continued)

Compound	Odor description	Odor threshold (ppm v/v)	Refs
Thiocyanic acid (2)			(2)
Ethanethioic acid-S-ME (2)			(2)
Methylbenzotiophene (2)			(2)
Benzenecarbothiotic acid (2)			(2)
Methanesulfonylazide (2)			(2)
Dimethyl sulfide	Cabbage	0.0030	**(4, 5)**
Allyl methyl sulfide			(4, 10)
Allyl isothiocyanate			(10)
Diallyl disulfide			(6)
Hydrogen sulfide	Rotten egg	0.00041	**(4)**
Methyl mercaptan	Sewer	0.000070	**(2, 4)**
Dimethyldisulfide	Sulfur	0.0022	**(1, 2, 4, 5)**
Dimethyltrisulfide	–	–	**(1, 2, 4, 5)**

(1) Kostelc et al. (1980); (2) Claus et al. (1996); (3) Cooke et al. (2003); (4) van den Velde et al. (2007); (5) Van den Velde et al. (2009); (6) Ross et al. (2009); (7) Goldberg et al. (1994); (8) Amano et al. (2002); (9) Berg et al. (1946); (10) Al-Kateb et al. (2013). ($N = 83$ compounds). Compounds that have been associated with breath odors are written in boldface. Methenamine is produced by the reaction of formaldehyde and ammonia (Van den Velde et al. 2009)

significant correlations comparing odor levels with cadaverine (Goldberg et al. 1994) and ammonia (Amano et al. 2002).

These results, taken together with clinical experience, may suggest that breath odors are more complex, and in fact are composed a "bouquet" of many different volatiles. This may explain the different types and characteristics of breath odors, and the observation that in certain individual's odor does not correlate with one or more measured component. The technical difficulties in measuring some of the malodor components such as low instrumental sensitivity or the inability of a method to detect certain compounds may also play a part in underestimating the role of various breath malodor components.

3.5 Microbial Aspects

3.5.1 Malodor-Producing Microorganisms

Much like other bacterial associated ailments in the oral cavity (e.g., caries and periodontal disease), there is an ongoing dispute among researchers as to whether oral malodor is caused by specific bacteria (specific theory), various types of bacteria sharing the same metabolic processes (nonspecific theory), or simply an over-

growth of the entire bacterial population (bacterial load).

Early observations suggested that malodor production is a complex process. In 1946, Berg and Fosdick (1946) tested the ability of 17 oral microorganisms to putrefy saliva and increase malodor production following aerobic and anaerobic incubation. They found that although all of the microorganisms caused some increase in salivary putrefaction, it was evident that no single type of organism was capable of putrefying saliva as rapidly as the mixtures normally present in the mouth.

Research also demonstrated that the putrefaction process was accompanied by a shift in the bacterial composition of the incubation mixture. Shiota and Kunkel (1958) showed that in incubated whole saliva there was a decrease over time in the streptococci and lactobacilli populations, whereas fusiforms, pH, indole, and ammonia levels increased. These processes were inhibited when the saliva was incubated in the presence of glucose. In this instance, streptococci and lactobacilli populations increased concomitant with a decrease in pH.

Subsequent research provided further evidence that the Gram-negative bacterial population was directly responsible for malodor production in vitro. McNamara and colleagues (1972) showed that inoculation of liquid incubation medium with Gram-negative oral bacteria, but not Gram-positive resulted in malodor production. Furthermore, they showed that incubating whole saliva resulted in a bacterial shift from a predominantly Gram-positive population to a predominantly Gram-negative one. This shift was accompanied with malodor production and rise in pH. They also showed that the addition of glucose-inhibited malodor production while maintaining Gram-positive predominance. Kleinberg and Codipilly (1997) also showed that incubating pure bacterial cultures of Gram-negative oral bacteria species such as *Fusobacterium, Porphyromonas,* and *Prevotella* in the presence of various free amino acids resulted in malodor production whereas Gram-positive (*Streptococci, Actinomyces,* and *lactobacilli*) did not.

In order to evaluate whether specific types of bacteria are involve in oral malodor production, bacterial samples were taken from the tongue dorsum of individuals with and without oral malodor and identified using molecular techniques (e.g., PCR; polymerized chain reaction), thus allowing the identification of both cultivable and non-cultivable bacteria (Haraszthy et al. 2007; Kazor et al. 2003; Riggio et al. 2008). Despite the great variation between subjects reported by all the researchers, few bacteria seemed to be unique to the oral malodor positive patients. These are specified in Table 3.5.

All three studies reported greater bacterial diversity in oral malodor-positive subjects, and a difference in the proportions of bacterial population in each group was also noted. Interestingly, all these studies reported *Solobacterium moorei*, a Gram-positive bacterium, to be prevalent on the tongue dorsum of malodor-positive subjects.

Despite the fact that two of these studies found *S. salivarius* prevalent in all the subjects (Haraszthy et al. 2007; Riggio et al. 2008), one study reported it to be found mostly in oral malodor negative subjects (Kazor et al. 2003). However, careful examination of the data reveals that the subjects from the malodor-positive group who did habor this bacterium showed distinctively higher levels of volatile sulfides and malodor. Interestingly, in one of the studies

Table 3.5 Bacteria associated with malodor from tongue dorsum

Solobacterium (Bulleidia) moorei	1, 2, 3
Granulicatella elegans	2, 3
Granulicatella adiacens	3
Eubacterium species	1, 2, 3
Firmicutes species	2
Porphyromonas species	2
Staphylococcus warneri	2
Dialister species	1, 2
Prevotella intermedia	2
Prevotella pallens	3
Prevotella shahii	3
Prevotella tannerae	3
Uncultured Prevotella sp.	3
Atopobium parvulum	1
Fusobacterium periodonticum	1
Fusobacterium sulci	3
Streptococcus phylotype (clone BW009)	1
Phylum TM7 phylotype (clone DR034)	1
Cryptobacterium curtum	1
Bacteroides forsythus (Tannerella forsythensis)	3
Capnocytophaga gingivalis	3
Capnocytophaga sputigena	3
Escherichia coli	3
Gemella haemolysans	3
Gemella sanguinis	3
Lachnospiraceae bacterium	3
Megasphaera sp. oral clone	3
Mogibacterium neglectum	3
Neisseria perflava	3
Neisseria subflava	3
Rothia dentocariosa	3
Streptococcus australis	3
Streptococcus cristatus	3
Uncultured Streptococcus sp.	3

(1) Kazor et al. (2003); (2) Haraszthy et al. (2007); (3) Riggio et al. (2008)

(Haraszthy et al. 2007), *Fusobacterium nucleatum*, a putative malodor-producing Gram-negative oral bacterium, was also present in all the malodor-negative subjects.

Studies conducted on the bacteria of periodontal pockets aimed to identify the malodor associated bacteria are summarized in Table 3.6.

Although some overlapping between malodor-producing bacteria from periodontal pockets and tongue dorsum can be seen (e.g., *Eubacterium, Fusobacterium,* and *Prevotella* species), some species (e.g., *Treponema, Bacteroides,* and *Porphyromonas*) appear to be more highly asso-

Table 3.6 Bacteria associated with malodor from periodontal pockets

Prevotella intermedia	1, 2
Prevotella nigrescens	2
Bacteroides forsythus	1, 2
Fusobacterium periodonticum	2
Fusobacterium nucleatum ss nucleatum	1, 2
Fusobacterium nucleatum ss vincentii	2
Fusobacterium nucleatum ss polymorphum	2
Treponema denticola	1, 2
Treponema socranskii	2
Porphyromonas gingivalis	1, 2
Campylobacter rectus	2
Campylobacter gracilis	2
Capnocytophaga ochracea	2
Capnocytophaga gingivalis	2
Eubacterium nodatum	1, 2
Selenomonas noxia	2
Propionibacterium acnes	2
Leptotrichia buccalis	2

(1) Persson et al. (1990); (2) Torresyap et al. (2003)

ciated with malodor exuding from periodontal pockets.

Persson and coworkers (1990) demonstrated the ability of certain periopathogenic bacteria (e.g., *Fusobacterium, Bacteroides,* and *Porphyromonas*) sampled from deep periodontal pockets to produce volatile sulfide compounds.

Some studies detected periopathogenic bacteria (*P. gingivalis, Tannerella forsythia, Prevotella intermedia, Prevotella nigrescens,* and *Treponema denticola*) in tongue-coating samples of subjects with oral malodor (Kato et al. 2005; Kurata et al. 2008; Tanaka et al. 2004). However, the prevalence of these bacteria was significantly higher in subjects who showed signs of periodontal disease (i.e., pocket depth of 4 mm and above) and higher in subgingival plaque as compared to tongue coating and saliva (Kato et al. 2005). Furthermore, the prevalence of these periopathogenic species in tongue-coating samples correlated with the tongue coating thickness (rather than area) and volatile sulfide levels, but showed only poor correlations with malodor scores (Tanaka et al. 2004). Interestingly, the improvement in periodontal health and oral VSC resulting from periodontal therapy did not seemed to affect the prevalence of periodontal pathogens in the tongue coating (Kurata et al. 2008). This

raised the possibility that periodontal pathogens residing on the tongue may serve as a reservoir for infection and reinfection of the periodontium.

Other studies have taken a different approach to studying the tongue dorsum microbial differences between subjects with or without oral malodor. Rather than identifying specific bacteria, they relied on their biochemical properties, by quantifying the levels of bacteria that are able to produce hydrogen sulfide (Hartley et al. 1996; Washio et al. 2005) as well as evaluating the total bacterial load. Both studies reported an increase in bacterial load associated with oral malodor as well as an increase in the amount of hydrogen sulfide-producing bacteria. However, whereas one study reported that the proportions of hydrogen sulfide producing bacteria were higher in the oral malodor positive group (Hartley et al. 1996), the other found no difference in their proportion between groups (Washio et al. 2005).

Recent developments in the field of molecular microbiology such as the Human Oral Microbiome Database (Dewhirst et al. 2010) and the use of deep sequencing techniques have opened up new pathways for understanding the complex microbial population (i.e., oral microbiome) of the oral cavity in health and disease. The observation that different niches in the oral cavity are populated by different bacterial species suggests that the oral microbiome is not a single entity but comprises different subpopulations. This in turn underlies the importance of site-specific intraoral sampling with regard to certain conditions. For example, whereas a study conducted on children with or without oral malodor using deep sequencing of supragingival samples did not find significant differences between groups (Ren et al. 2016a), another study done by the same research group using samples taken from tongue and saliva did (Ren et al. 2016b). Although, some differences in the abundance of certain bacterial genus and species were noted between malodorous and non-malodorous samples using this new methodology its main contribution, however, is to provide a broader view of the microbial ecosystem. To this effect, recent results have shown a higher microbial diversity as well as clustering of microbial profiles in malodorous samples as compared with non-malodorous ones (Yitzhaki et al. 2018).

Most studies carried out on the microbial aspect of oral malodor report great variation in bacterial populations among individual subjects. Given the large prevalence of this condition, it is thus unlikely that only a few types of bacteria are involved. Nevertheless, specific microbial factors appear to contribute strongly to malodor production. It seems that microbial overgrowth (e.g., microbial load) as reflected mainly by tongue biofilm thickness and subgingival plaque accumulation is a key factor in oral malodor. The accumulation and thickening of the oral biofilms allow for the depletion of oxygen in the deep layers of the biofilm and the creation of anaerobic niches. Whether or not this process is accompanied by a change in the proportion of the various types of bacteria (floral shift), or an increase in bacterial diversity, the overall bacterial activity leads to putrefactive action in the oral cavity which is the underlying cause of malodor production.

References

Al-Kateb H, de Lacy CB, Ratcliffe N. An investigation of volatile organic compounds from the saliva of healthy individuals using headspace-trap/GC-MS. J Breath Res. 2013;7(3):036004.

Amano A, Yoshida Y, Oho T, Koga T. Monitoring ammonia to assess halitosis. Oral Surg Oral Med Oral Pathol Oral Radiol Endod. 2002;94(6):692–6.

Berg M, Fosdick LS. Studies in periodontal disease: II. Putrefactive organisms in the mouth. J Dent Res. 1946;25:73–81.

Berg M, Burrill DY, Fosdick LS. Chemical studies in periodontal disease III: putrefaction of salivary proteins. J Dent Res. 1946;25:231–46.

Claus D, Geypens B, Rutgeerts P, Ghyselen J, Hoshi K, Van Steenberghe D, Ghoos Y. Where gastroenterology and periodontology meets: determination of oral volatile organic compounds using closed loop trapping and high resolution gas chromatography ion trap detection. In: Van Steenberghe D, Rosenberg M, editors. Bad breath a multidisciplinary approach. Leuven: Leuven University Press; 1996. p. 15–27.

Codipilly DP, Kaufman HW, Kleinberg I. Use of a novel group of oral malodor measurements to evaluate an anti-oral malodor mouthrinse (TriOralTM) in humans. J Clin Dent. 2004;15(4):98–104.

Cooke M, Leeves N, White C. Time profile of putrescine, cadaverine, indole and skatole in human saliva. Arch Oral Biol. 2003;48(4):323–7.

Dewhirst FE, Chen T, Izard J, Paster BJ, Tanner AC, Yu WH, Lakshmanan A, Wade WG. The human oral microbiome. J Bacteriol. 2010;192(19):5002–17.

Fosdick LS, Piez KA. Chemical studies in periodontal disease. X. Paper chromatographic investigation of the putrefaction associated with periodontitis. J Dent Res. 1953;32(1):87–100.

Gochman N, Meyer RK, Blackwell RQ, Fosdick LS. The amino acid decarboxylase of salivary sediment. J Dent Res. 1959;38:998–1003.

Goldberg S, Kozlovsky A, Gordon D, Gelernter I, Sintov A, Rosenberg M. Cadaverine as a putative component of oral malodor. J Dent Res. 1994;73(6):1168–72.

Greenstein RB, Goldberg S, Marku-Cohen S, Sterer N, Rosenberg M. Reduction of oral malodor by oxidizing lozenges. J Periodontol. 1997;68(12):1176–81.

Haraszthy VI, Zambon JJ, Sreenivasan PK, Zambon MM, Gerber D, Rego R, Parker C. Identification of oral bacterial species associated with halitosis. J Am Dent Assoc. 2007;138(8):1113–20.

Hartley MG, El Maaytah MA, McKenzie C, Greenman J. The tongue microbiota of low odour and malodourous individuals. Microbial Ecol Health Dis. 1996;9:215–23.

Kato H, Yoshida A, Awano S, Ansai T, Takehara T. Quantitative detection of volatile sulfur compound-producing microorganisms in oral specimens using real-time PCR. Oral Dis. 2005;11(Suppl 1):67–71.

Kazor CE, Mitchell PM, Lee AM, Stokes LN, Loesche WJ, Dewhirst FE, Paster BJ. Diversity of bacterial populations on the tongue dorsa of patients with halitosis and healthy patients. J Clin Microbiol. 2003;41(2):558–63.

Kleinberg I, Codipilly DM. The biological basis of oral malodor formation. In: Rosenberg M, editor. Bad breath: research perspectives. Tel Aviv: Ramot publishing Tel Aviv University; 1997. p. 13–39.

Kleinberg I, Wolff MS, Codipilly DM. Role of saliva in oral dryness, oral feel and oral malodour. Int Dent J. 2002;52(Suppl 3):236–40.

Kostelc JG, Preti G, Zelson PR, Stoller NH, Tonzetich J. Salivary volatiles as indicators of periodontitis. J Periodontal Res. 1980;15(2):185–92.

Kurata H, Awano S, Yoshida A, Ansai T, Takehara T. The prevalence of periodontopathogenic bacteria in saliva is linked to periodontal health status and oral malodour. J Med Microbiol. 2008;57(Pt 5):636–42.

Mackie RI, Stroot PG, Varel VH. Biochemical identification and biological origin of key odor components in livestock waste. J Anim Sci. 1998;76(5):1331–42.

McNamara TF, Alexander JF, Lee M. The role of microorganisms in the production of oral malodor. Oral Surg Oral Med Oral Pathol. 1972;34(1):41–8.

Persson S, Edlund MB, Claesson R, Carlsson J. The formation of hydrogen sulfide and methyl mercaptan by oral bacteria. Oral Microbiol Immunol. 1990;5(4):195–201.

Ren W, Xun Z, Wang Z, Zhang Q, Liu X, Zheng H, Zhang Q, Zhang Y, Zhang L, Wu C, Zheng S, Qin N, Ehrlich SD, Li Y, He X, Xu T, Chen T, Chen F. Tongue coating and the salivary microbial communities vary in children with halitosis. Sci Rep. 2016a;6:24481.

Ren W, Zhang Q, Liu X, Zheng S, Ma L, Chen F, Xu T, Xu B. Supragingival plaque microbial community analysis of children with halitosis. J Microbiol Biotechnol. 2016b;26(12):2141–7.

Riggio MP, Lennon A, Rolph HJ, Hodge PJ, Donaldson A, Maxwell AJ, Bagg J. Molecular identification of bacteria on the tongue dorsum of subjects with and without halitosis. Oral Dis. 2008;14(3):251–8.

Ross BM, Dadgostar N, Bloom M, McKeown L. The analysis of oral air using selected ion flow tube mass spectrometry in persons with and without a history of oral malodour. Int J Dent Hyg. 2009;7(2):136–43.

Shiota T, Kunkel MF Jr. In vitro chemical and bacterial changes in saliva. J Dent Res. 1958;37(5):780–7.

Sterer N, Rosenberg M. *Streptococcus salivarius* promotes mucin putrefaction and malodor production by *Porphyromonas gingivalis*. J Dent Res. 2006;85(10):910–4.

Sterer N, Greenstein RB, Rosenberg M. Beta-galactosidase activity in saliva is associated with oral malodor. J Dent Res. 2002;81(3):182–5.

Sterer N, Shaharabany M, Rosenberg M. β-Galactosidase activity and H2S production in an experimental oral biofilm. J Breath Res. 2009;3(016006):4pp.

Tanaka M, Yamamoto Y, Kuboniwa M, Nonaka A, Nishida N, Maeda K, Kataoka K, Nagata H, Shizukuishi S. Contribution of periodontal pathogens on tongue dorsa analyzed with real-time PCR to oral malodor. Microbes Infect. 2004;6(12):1078–83.

Tonzetich J. Direct gas chromatographic analysis of sulphur compounds in mouth air in man. Arch Oral Biol. 1971;16(6):587–97.

Tonzetich J, Richter VJ. Evaluation of volatile odoriferous components of saliva. Arch Oral Biol. 1964;16:39–46.

Tonzetich J, Eigen E, King WJ, Weiss S. Volatility as a factor in the inability of certain amines and indole to increase the odour of saliva. Arch Oral Biol. 1967;12(10):1167–75.

Torresyap G, Haffajee AD, Uzel NG, Socransky SS. Relationship between periodontal pocket sulfide levels and subgingival species. J Clin Periodontol. 2003;30(11):1003–10.

van den Velde S, Quirynen M, van Hee P, van Steenberghe D. Halitosis associated volatiles in breath of healthy subjects. J Chromatogr B Analyt Technol Biomed Life Sci. 2007;853(1–2):54–61.

Van den Velde S, van Steenberghe D, Van Hee P, Quirynen M. Detection of odorous compounds in breath. J Dent Res. 2009;88(3):285–9.

Washio J, Sato T, Koseki T, Takahashi N. Hydrogen sulfide-producing bacteria in tongue biofilm and their relationship with oral malodour. J Med Microbiol. 2005;54(Pt 9):889–95.

Yitzhaki S, Reshef L, Gophna U, Rosenberg M, Sterer N. Microbiome associated with denture malodour. J Breath Res. 2018;12(2):027103.

Odor Perception

4

Contents

4.1   Olfactory Psychophysics

The sense of smell is the least understood of all human senses. The olfaction process is a complex one involving both physiological peripheral sensing and cognitive and emotional central processing. The olfactory receptor neurons are situated in the olfactory epithelium located in the upper portion of the nasal cavity. These cells project cilia into the mucus lining of the nasal cavity, and those are responsible for the first stages of the olfaction process. The binding of an odor molecule to the receptor results in an electrical signal that is transducted through the neuron's axon to the olfactory bulb, and causes the release of a neurotransmitter (Berkowicz et al. 1994) which activates mitral and tufted cells within the olfactory bulb to carry the information further into the brain. Within the brain, the olfactory system is closely linked to areas of the brain that are involved with emotion (i.e., Amygdala; Cain and Bindra 1972; Zald and Pardo 1997), memory, and learning (i.e., the hippocampus).

We do not yet completely understand which odorants activates a certain receptor. However, it seems that different combinations of olfactory neuron activation may have the potential to explain the large variety of detectible odors. Research has shown that different receptors families are expressed zonally across the olfactory epithelium (Strotmann et al. 1994), which coincides with zones of odorant sensitivity. This may suggest that odor qualities are coded at the level of the olfactory bulb on the basis of distributed patterns of activity (Shepherd 1994).

Genetic variations in human odorant receptors may account for the vast differences in odor perception between different individuals (Keller et al. 2007). Furthermore, genetic differences in receptor expression may help to explain why some individuals with a normal sense of smell may be "blinded" to a single odorant or a small group of closely related odorant (i.e., specific anosmia; Amoore 1977). However, repeated exposure to an odorant did seem to induce the ability to detect it by subject who were initially anosmic to it (Dorries et al. 1989).

© Springer Nature Switzerland AG 2020

N. Sterer, M. Rosenberg, *Breath Odors*, https://doi.org/10.1007/978-3-030-44731-1_4

Research has shown that a certain amount of electrical activity is always present in the olfactory neurons. This activity is referred to as baseline "noise" (Cain 1977), and is considered to increase olfaction sensitivity on the expense of specificity. This implies that the receptors are easily activated by minute concentration of odorants even with marginal odorant–receptor fit.

The response to a certain odorant is terminated, presumably to allow the system to be ready for the next stimulus. This process (i.e., adaptation) occurs both peripherally at the receptor cell and centrally in the brain. At the receptor cell level, olfactory adaptation is calcium-dependent (Kurahashi and Menini 1997); therefore, this process may be affected by medications or conditions that affect cellular calcium homeostasis. Central adaptation mechanism is not yet understood. However, unlike receptor cell adaptation that is considered short-term (minutes), central adaptation may last for as long as 4 weeks (Dalton and Wysocki 1996).

Various diseases and conditions may affect olfactory function. For example, research has shown that the neurotransmitter dopamine decreases the baseline activity (i.e., "noise") of mitral cells in the olfactory bulb (Duchamp-Viret et al. 1997). Therefore, in patients with Parkinson's disease in which dopamine synthesis is impaired, the ability to identify odors may be reduced (Doty et al. 1991). These patients' olfactory disorder was shown to be independent of the cognitive, perceptual–motor, and memory manifestations of the disease (Doty et al. 1989). The rich cortical representation of the olfactory system on all its various components contributes to the normal function of odor perception and memory. This complexity, however, makes it sensitive to pathology and disease. Odor perception may be impaired by various disorders such as Alzheimer's disease, schizophrenia, depression, autism, and early life exposure to toxins, while other sensory systems remain for the most part unaffected (Wilson et al. 2014).

Most studies conducted on the relationship between gender and olfaction have concluded that at least for some odorants, females perform better than males in odor detection, identifica-

tion, and discrimination (Doty and Cameron 2009). Estrogen modulates the activity of retinoic acid, an important factor in olfactory cells differentiation (Balboni et al. 1991). This might explain the observation that premenopause females tend to perform better than males in olfactory function tests (Wysocki and Gilbert 1989). However, a recent systematic review that examined the data about sex hormone alterations (e.g., menstrual cycle, pregnancy, gonadectomy, and hormone replacement therapy) and human olfactory function concluded that the relationship between the two is complex and any simple explanation for any association between them is tenuous (Doty and Cameron 2009). One recent study showed that females of three different age groups (19–39, 40–59, >60) performed significantly better than males for both odor threshold and odor discrimination, thus demonstrating higher olfactory sensitivity (Thuerauf et al. 2009). The researchers attributed this to the link between odors and emotional reactivity, since females demonstrated better emotion-linked memory (Canli et al. 2002).

Cognitive factors have been shown to impact human odor perception. Research showed that subjects who were given a negative description of an odor gave higher intensity scores, perceived it as irritating, and were less adaptive to it than those who were given a neutral or positive description (Dalton et al. 1997). Learning and memory also play a strong part in odor perception. Our familiarity and associated experience with a certain odorant will affect the way that we classify its pleasantness. Furthermore, it seems that odor perception is highly linked to emotional state, which effects both odor identification and intensity ratings (Hoenen et al. 2017).

Taken together these physiological and environmental factors may help to explain the high intra and interindividual variability seen in psychophysical research on olfactory threshold (Stevens et al. 1988).

Nevertheless, it seems that some level of consensus may be associated to various chemical traits of certain odorants. In a study conducted on the verbal description of 480 different molecules by 55 subjects (Keller and Vosshall 2016), one of the findings most relevant to the topic of breath odors suggested that the number of sulfur atoms in a molecule was in correlation with odor descriptors such as "garlic," "fish," and "decayed." It is possible that through our evolution we have come to recognize some chemicals as a warning sign in order to avoid the ingestion of spoiled foods and polluted water sources.

4.2   Odor Mixtures

Naturally occurring smells such as breath odors are usually a complex mixture of various odorants. Unlike some other sensory systems in which the intensity of a complex signal is the sum of its components (i.e., additivity), in olfaction this rule does not seem to apply. Studies done on two component mixtures show that in most cases, mixing the odorants results in the suppression of the perceived intensity of one or both odors (Laing et al. 1984). Although the strength of an odor may be increased by the presence of another (i.e., synergism), this is rarely seen in two component mixtures. However, some researchers have reported a substantial synergistic effect in a complex mixture of many odorants (Laska and Hudson 1991) at concentration too low to be sensed individually (i.e., subthreshold).

Some studies have been conducted on the interactions of unpleasant odor components (Berglund 1974). These studies showed that the odor intensity of two, three, and four component mixtures of volatile sulfides (hydrogen sulfide, dimethylsulfide, dimethyldisulfide, and methylmercaptan) slightly exceeded the intensity of the single odorants. Another more recent study (Laing et al. 1994) conducted on odor interactions of malodorous components (hydrogen sulfide, butanethiol, skatol, and isovaleric acid) concluded that suppression was the dominant perceptual effect. It also concluded that there was a substantial loss of identity of the individual odorants in the mixture, a finding that is in agreement with other studies which demonstrated that humans have considerable difficulty in identifying three or four odorants in a given mixture (Laing and Francis 1989). Interestingly, it seems that the malodor of the mixture was usually perceived as more unpleasant than any of the individual components (Laing et al. 1994). This suggested that the loss of odorant identity was not mostly due to the reduced odor intensity of the component but rather due to the blending of one or more of the components to produce an even fouler smell (Laing et al. 1994).

4.3   Odor Perception and Odor Evaluation Panels

Organoleptic scores given by odor judges are the most common means of evaluating a malodor nuisance and are considered as the golden standard in breath odor investigations. However, given the large interpersonal variation in odor perception, using a panel of several evaluators is recommended.

Studies conducted on the implementation of odor perception principals on the accuracy and repeatability of organoleptic (odor judge) measurements stress the importance of proper panel selection and training techniques. For example, it was suggested that using varying concentration of odorant samples (i.e., n-butanol) in a double blind manner was less repetitive and more effective than the standard one concentration method (Capelli et al. 2010). Although olfactory memory seems to be linked to the experience of the panelists in recognizing the measured malodor (i.e., stimulus familiarity), trained panelists were shown to be more accurate than nontrained (naive) ones regardless of their level of familiarity. However, panel experience did allow the trained panelists to verbalize their perception more accurately when the stimuli were familiar (Lesschaeve and Issanchou 1996).

Rosenberg and coworkers (1991) found that inter-examiner correlations among judges with no prior experience in scoring breath odors were mostly significant with r values ranging from 0.14 to 0.49.

Other researchers have also reported that training improves the accuracy of odor intensity scoring by both experienced and inexperienced panelists (Nachnani et al. 2005). Interestingly, training did not seem to improve the ability to discriminate and identify different odorants in a mixture (Livermore and Laing 1996).

Researchers who studied the relationship between oral malodor intensity scale and the concentration of some of its components (e.g., hydrogen sulfide, skatole, cadaverine) suggested that the intensity score reflects the odorant–receptor binding ratio (e.g., increasing saturation), which is logarithmic in nature and depends on the odor threshold and odor power (i.e., the ratio between odor score and concentration) of each odorant (Greenman et al. 2005). Understanding that the organoleptic oral malodor intensity scale is indeed an exponential scale may enable the design of better ways to train and calibrate the odor judge panel.

References

Amoore JE. Specific anosmia and the concept of primary odors. Chem Senses Flavour. 1977;2:267–81.

Balboni GC, Zonefrati R, Repice F, Barni T, Vannelli GB. Immunohistochemical detection of EGF and NGF receptors in human olfactory epithelium. Boll Soc Ital Biol Sper. 1991;67(10–11):901–6.

Berglund B. Quantitative and qualitative analysis of industrial odors with human observers. Ann N Y Acad Sci. 1974;237(0):35–51.

Berkowicz DA, Trombley PQ, Shepherd GM. Evidence for glutamate as the olfactory receptor cell neurotransmitter. J Neurophysiol. 1994;71(6):2557–61.

Cain WS. Differential sensitivity for smell: "noise" at the nose. Science. 1977;195(4280):796–8.

Cain DP, Bindra D. Responses of amygdala single units to odors in the rat. Exp Neurol. 1972;35(1):98–110.

Canli T, Desmond JE, Zhao Z, Gabrieli JD. Sex differences in the neural basis of emotional memories. Proc Natl Acad Sci U S A. 2002;99(16):10789–94.

Capelli L, Sironi S, Del Rosso R, Centola P, Bonati S. Improvement of olfactometric measurement accuracy and repeatability by optimization of panel selection procedures. Water Sci Technol. 2010;61(5):1267–78.

Dalton P, Wysocki CJ. The nature and duration of adaptation following long-term odor exposure. Percept Psychophys. 1996;58(5):781–92.

Dalton P, Wysocki CJ, Brody MJ, Lawley HJ. The influence of cognitive bias on the perceived odor, irritation and health symptoms from chemical exposure. Int Arch Occup Environ Health. 1997;69(6):407–17.

Dorries KM, Schmidt HJ, Beauchamp GK, Wysocki CJ. Changes in sensitivity to the odor of androstenone during adolescence. Dev Psychobiol. 1989;22(5):423–35.

Doty RL, Cameron EL. Sex differences and reproductive hormone influences on human odor perception. Physiol Behav. 2009;97(2):213–28.

Doty RL, Riklan M, Deems DA, Reynolds C, Stellar S. The olfactory and cognitive deficits of Parkinson's disease: evidence for independence. Ann Neurol. 1989;25(2):166–71.

Doty RL, Perl DP, Steele JC, Chen KM, Pierce JD Jr, Reyes P, Kurland LT. Olfactory dysfunction in three neurodegenerative diseases. Geriatrics. 1991;46(Suppl 1):47–51.

Duchamp-Viret P, Coronas V, Delaleu JC, Moyse E, Duchamp A. Dopaminergic modulation of mitral cell activity in the frog olfactory bulb: a combined radioligand binding-electrophysiological study. Neuroscience. 1997;79(1):203–16.

Greenman J, El-Maaytah M, Duffield J, Spencer P, Rosenberg M, Corry D, Saad S, Lenton P, Majerus G, Nachnani S. Assessing the relationship between concentrations of malodor compounds and odor scores from judges. J Am Dent Assoc. 2005;136(6):749–57.

Hoenen M, Wolf OT, Pause BM. The impact of stress on odor perception. Perception. 2017;46(3–4):366–76.

Keller A, Vosshall LB. Olfactory perception of chemically diverse molecules. BMC Neurosci. 2016;17(1):55.

Keller A, Zhuang H, Chi Q, Vosshall LB, Matsunami H. Genetic variation in a human odorant receptor alters odour perception. Nature. 2007;449(7161):468–72.

Kurahashi T, Menini A. Mechanism of odorant adaptation in the olfactory receptor cell. Nature. 1997;385(6618):725–9.

Laing DG, Francis GW. The capacity of humans to identify odors in mixtures. Physiol Behav. 1989;46(5):809–14.

Laing DG, Panhuber H, Willcox ME, Pittman EA. Quality and intensity of binary odor mixtures. Physiol Behav. 1984;33(2):309–19.

Laing DG, Eddy A, Best DJ. Perceptual characteristics of binary, trinary, and quaternary odor mixtures consisting of unpleasant constituents. Physiol Behav. 1994;56(1):81–93.

Laska M, Hudson R. A comparison of the detection thresholds of odour mixtures and their components. Chem Senses. 1991;16(6):651–62.

Lesschaeve I, Issanchou S. Effects of panel experience on olfactory memory performance: influence of stimuli familiarity and labeling ability of subjects. Chem Senses. 1996;21(6):699–709.

Livermore A, Laing DG. Influence of training and experience on the perception of multicomponent odor mixtures. J Exp Psychol Hum Percept Perform. 1996;22(2):267–77.

Nachnani S, Majerus G, Lenton P, Hodges J, Magallanes E. Effects of training on odor judges scoring intensity. Oral Dis. 2005;11(Suppl 1):40–4.

Rosenberg M, Septon I, Eli I, Bar-Ness R, Gelernter I, Brenner S, Gabbay J. Halitosis measurement by an industrial sulphide monitor. J Periodontol. 1991;62(8):487–9.

Shepherd GM. Discrimination of molecular signals by the olfactory receptor neuron. Neuron. 1994;13(4):771–90.

Stevens JC, Cain WS, Burke RJ. Variability of olfactory thresholds. Chem Senses. 1988;13:643–53.

Strotmann J, Wanner I, Helfrich T, Beck A, Meinken C, Kubick S, Breer H. Olfactory neurones expressing distinct odorant receptor subtypes are spatially segregated in the nasal neuroepithelium. Cell Tissue Res. 1994;276(3):429–38.

Thuerauf N, Reulbach U, Lunkenheimer J, Lunkenheimer B, Spannenberger R, Gossler A, Maihofner C, Bleich S, Kornhuber J, Markovic K. Emotional reactivity to odors: olfactory sensitivity and the span of emotional evaluation separate the genders. Neurosci Lett. 2009;456(2):74–9.

Wilson DA, Xu W, Sadrian B, Courtiol E, Cohen Y, Barnes DC. Cortical odor processing in health and disease. Prog Brain Res. 2014;208:275–305.

Wysocki CJ, Gilbert AN. National Geographic Smell Survey. Effects of age are heterogenous. Ann N Y Acad Sci. 1989;561:12–28.

Zald DH, Pardo JV. Emotion, olfaction, and the human amygdala: amygdala activation during aversive olfactory stimulation. Proc Natl Acad Sci U S A. 1997;94(8):4119–24.

Breath Odors of Nasal and Pharyngeal Origin

Contents

According to reports from various multidisciplinary breath odor clinics around the world, some 4–8% of breath odor cases are ear–nose–throat (ENT)-related conditions (Quirynen et al. 2009; Seemann et al. 2006). These include nasal and pharyngeal infections and conditions such as chronic sinusitis, chronic (caseous) tonsillitis, foreign bodies, and craniofacial anomalies (e.g., cleft palate). These are specified in Table 5.1.

5.1 Chronic Sinusitis

The sinuses are drained and ventilated into the nasal cavity through small orifices (i.e., ostium). Any obstruction in the sinuses' drainage resulting from malformation or disease may cause sinus secretion stagnation and bacterial infection (Stammberger 1986). This condition differs from acute sinusitis in its symptoms, which are mostly related to an increase in nasal secretions (i.e., postnasal drip). These include chronic cough, productive throat cleaning, sniffling, and halitosis (Bunzen et al. 2006; Tatli et al. 2001). Furthermore, Gram-negative anaerobic bacteria (e.g., Bacteroides sp. and Fusobacteria sp.) that are known producers of VSC have been shown to inhabit the maxillary sinuses (Brook 1981).

In those cases in which the breath odor results from a nasal infection the malodor is typically felt much stronger from the air exhaled through the nose (Rosenberg 1996). However, it is important to stress that postnasal drip may be an important factor in tongue malodor (Rosenberg and Leib 1997); therefore, an additional oral malodor component is expected to be present in cases of chronic sinusitis.

The diagnosis of chronic sinusitis is best confirmed by an otolaryngologic examination using a flexible endoscope (Finkelstein 1997a). The flexible endoscope allows the clinician to examine the areas of inflammation or pathologic drainage in the intranasal structures, which cannot otherwise be detected using anterior rhinoscopy

Table 5.1   ENT-related breath odor-inducing conditions

Pathology	Signs and symptoms	Diagnosis	Recommended treatment
Chronic rhinosinusitis	Nasal malodor Post nasal drip (PND)	Flexible endoscopy of the nasal cavity	Functional endoscopic sinus surgery (FESS)
Chronic caseous tonsillitis	Occasional oral malodor Tonsilloliths	Tonsils smelling test	CO_2 laser cryptolysis
Foreign bodies	Nasal malodor (unilateral) Purulent unilateral nasal discharge	Anterior rhinoscopy and flexible endoscopy of the nasal cavity	Foreign body extraction
Craniofacial anomalies	Nasal and oral malodor Cleft palate	Clinical examination	Corrective surgery

or plain sinus radiographs. In a study conducted on 275 children between the ages of 2 and 14 years (58% males), 67% of the children with a confirmed diagnosis of chronic rhinosinusitis showed signs of halitosis as compared with only 28% in the control (Leo et al. 2015).

Functional endoscopic sinus surgery (FESS) is currently a preferred treatment for chronic rhinosinusitis. In a retrospective clinical study carried out in Brazil on patients suffering from chronic rhinosinusitis (Bunzen et al. 2006), it was shown that in 10 out of 24 patients (41.6%) who initially complained of halitosis 8 reported improvement following this procedure.

5.2   Chronic Caseous Tonsillitis

The tonsils contain tubular invaginations known as crypts which extend from the tonsils' surface to deep within its parenchyma (Finkelstein et al. 2004). In some cases, caseous secretions may be retained within these crypts resulting in caseous tonsillitis that is considered a variant of chronic tonsillitis. This condition is characterized by the formation of calcareous concretions known as tonsilloliths or tonsillar calculi (Finkelstein et al. 2004).

Early clinical observations (Castellani 1930) suggested that this type of chronic tonsillitis (which they termed granulomycosis of the crypts) may be a cause for halitosis (i.e., fetor oris). These researchers noticed that "*in certain cases of granulomycosis a most offensive odour is emitted when the granules are extracted and squashed.*" They further noticed that these granules contained a large variety of bacteria, and

were even able to isolate and grow certain Gram-negative bacilli "*which produce in agar culture exactly the same offensive odour as was noticeable in the patient's breath, and on squashing the white granules.*"

A more recent study on the microbial composition of tonsilloliths from six individuals conducted using culture-independent molecular methods (i.e., PCR), demonstrated the presence of many anaerobic bacterial species (Tsuneishi et al. 2006). These included *Eubacterium, Fusobacterium, Megasphaera, Porphyromonas, Prevotella, Selenomonas,* and *Tannerella*, all of which are associated with VSC production.

Chronic tonsillitis-associated malodor seems to occur intermittently (Fletcher and Blair 1988) and may be concomitant with the appearance and exfoliation of the tonsilloliths. Research showed that patients suffering from chronic caseous tonsillitis had a significantly higher VSC levels when tonsilloliths were present (Rio et al. 2008). Furthermore, one case reported in Japan showed that VSC readings sharply decreased following tonsilloliths removal (Kato et al. 2005).

Tonsil-associated malodor does not respond to standard oral care treatments (Talebian et al. 2008). Therefore, once intraoral origins have been ruled out and the malodor persists, especially if the malodor coincides with the appearance of tonsilloliths, then the tonsils are a likely source of the malodor.

In the past, halitosis of tonsillar origin was considered a valid indication for adenotonsillectomy (Arnold 1953). However, since then a more conservative method of treatment has been applied. This method, termed laser cryptolysis (Finkelstein et al. 2004) or laser cryptolysis by coagulation

(Rio et al. 2008), is aimed at opening the crypts ostium, thus preventing caseum retention. This procedure is carried out using CO_2 laser under local anesthesia. Research demonstrated that patients suffering from chronic caseous tonsillitis showed significant reduction in VSC levels following this treatment (Rio et al. 2008). Another study conducted on 34 patients suffering from caseous-related halitosis were treated using radiofrequency cryptolysis reported a 76% success rate in eliminating the problem in a 12 months follow-up as determined organoleptically (Ata et al. 2014).

5.3 Foreign Bodies

Young children typically 2–4 years of age tend to insert small objects such as plastic beads, buttons, and small toy parts into their nostrils (Kiger et al. 2008). This type of behavior usually ceases after the age of 5, although it may continue in older children (e.g. 10 or 11 years of age) in cases of attention-deficit hyperactivity disorder (ADHD; Perera et al. 2009), or at any age in cases of severe mental retardation (Rosenberg and Leib 1997).

In many cases, these foreign objects consist of plastic, cotton, organic matter, or paper, materials that would not normally appear in X-rays, and can only be detected using endoscopy (Fig. 5.1).

Typically, the chief complaint made by the child's parents at the doctor's office would refer to the child's severe body odor (Katz et al. 1979; Rosenberg and Leib 1997). However, a thorough clinical examination will usually reveal that the malodor is emanating from the nasal cavity (Rosenberg and Leib 1997) or the mouth (Syfert 1979). Upon examination a purulent inflammation of one nostril is noted accompanied by a

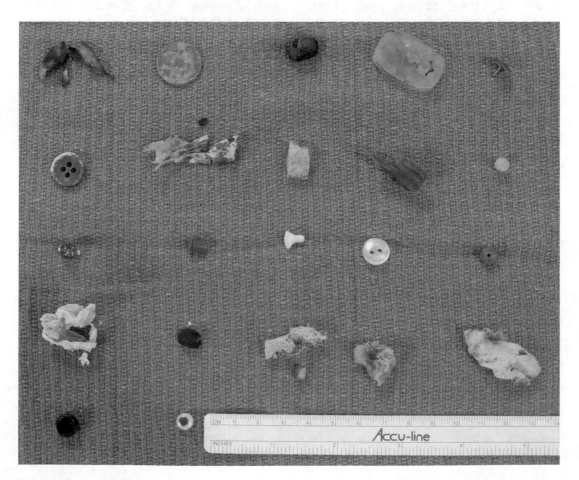

Fig. 5.1 Variety of foreign objects extracted from the nose of children (kindly provided by Dr. M. Marcus)

unilateral malodorous discharged from the same nostril. This smelly discharge is smeared by the child on his clothes and hair, therefore creating a mistaken impression of body odor (Syfert 1979). This can be verified by smelling areas on the child's body that are normally out of reach (e.g., back and ankles) that would not present the same malodor (Rosenberg and Leib 1997).

Nasal foreign bodies in children can usually be removed using simple techniques (Kiger et al. 2008). However, when left in place for years these objects may calcify over time creating a growing rhinolith (i.e., nasal stone) which may result in a unilateral nasal obstruction (Brehmer and Riemann 2010) in addition to the associated malodor. A case series study (Karli et al. 2012) conducted on eight female patients (age 14–45 years) showed that these rhinoliths were most commonly lodged between the middle and inferior concha and were associated with nasal obstruction (87%), purulent nasal discharge (75%), and malodor (37%).

Furthermore, although the nasal cavity is the most common site of breath odor causing foreign bodies, one case of a malodor causing pharyngeal foreign body was reported in the literature (Kurul and Kandogan 2002), suggesting that putrefying foreign objects may also be lodged in the pharynx.

In most cases of foreign bodies' related breath odor the malodor did not respond to antibiotic treatment. However, foreign body extraction results in immediate resolution of the foul odor.

5.4   Craniofacial Anomalies

Because of the various malformations in nasal structures observed in patients with craniofacial anomalies such as deviated nasal septum, deformed medial turbinate, underdeveloped maxillary sinuses, maxillary growth deficits, choanal stenosis or atresia, atresia of the nostrils, malformed external nasal valve, incompetent velopharyngeal valve, presence of pharyngeal flap and impairment of mucociliary transport, chronic paranasal sinusitis with accompanying breath odor formation is more frequently seen in patients with cleft palate (Finkelstein et al. 1990).

These structural malformations in the external and internal nasal passages may also cause nasal obstructions or high nasal airway resistance that may result in mouth breathing (Finkelstein 1997b), in itself a risk factor for oral malodor. Furthermore, poorer oral hygiene and dental condition have been observed in cases of cleft palate (Wong and King 1998). Both of these are also contributing factors to oral malodor formation. Finally, oronasal fistulas are often present in these patients and can serve as a continuous source of nasal contamination by oral bacteria. These fistulas may also facilitate the insertions of foreign bodies into the nasal cavity such as food or dental impression materials (Finkelstein 1997b).

Reports on breath odors in patients with craniofacial anomalies are mostly anecdotal case reports. However, a few clinical studies were published. One of these studies demonstrated no difference between the oral VSC levels of patients with repaired clefts and the control group (Monteiro-Amado et al. 2005), whereas a second study showed that both oral and nasal VSC levels were elevated in cleft patients especially in the affected nostril (Doruk et al. 2008). These results suggest that if malodor still persists following cleft repair then nasal malformations or infection should be examined next.

The above notwithstanding, much remains to be learnt about nasal malodor. Its characteristic odor is very different than that of oral malodor although both are attributed to anaerobic degradation of protein and amino acids. Furthermore, many cases of odor emanating from the nose appear to be unrelated to any frank medical condition.

References

Arnold JW. Controversial problems in adenotonsillectomy. Calif Med. 1953;78(5):444–9.

Ata N, Ovet G, Alataş N. Effectiveness of radiofrequency cryptolysis for the treatment of halitosis due to caseums. Am J Otolaryngol. 2014;35(2):93–8. https://doi.org/10.1016/j.amjoto.2013.11.010.

Brehmer D, Riemann R. The rhinolith—a possible differential diagnosis of a unilateral nasal obstruction. Case Rep Med 2010;2010(845671):4pp.

Brook I. Aerobic and anaerobic bacterial flora of normal maxillary sinuses. Laryngoscope. 1981;91(3):372–6.

Bunzen DL, Campos A, Leao FS, Morais A, Sperandio F, Caldas Neto S. Efficacy of functional endoscopic sinus surgery for symptoms in chronic rhinosinusitis with or without polyposis. Braz J Otorhinolaryngol. 2006;72(2):242–6. https://doi.org/10.1016/S1808-8694(15)30062-8.

Castellani A. Foetor oris of tonsillar origin and certain bacilli causing it. Lancet. 1930;22(March):623–4.

Doruk C, Ozturk F, Ozdemir H, Nalcaci R. Oral and nasal malodor in patients with and without cleft lip and palate who had undergone orthodontic therapy. Cleft Palate Craniofac J. 2008;45(5):481–4. https://doi.org/10.1597/07-074.1.

Finkelstein Y. The otolaryngologist and the patient with halitosis. In: Rosenberg M, editor. Bad breath research perspectives. Tel Aviv: Ramot Publishing—Tel Aviv University; 1997a. p. 175–87.

Finkelstein Y. Halitosis in patients with craniofacial anomalies. In: Rosenberg M, editor. Bad breath research perspectives. Tel Aviv: Ramot Publishing—Tel Aviv University; 1997b. p. 189–200.

Finkelstein Y, Talmi YP, Zohar Y. On the cause of sinusitis in patients with cleft palate. Arch Otolaryngol Head Neck Surg. 1990;116(4):490–1. https://doi.org/10.1001/archotol.1990.01870040112026.

Finkelstein Y, Talmi YP, Ophir D, Berger G. Laser cryptolysis for the treatment of halitosis. Otolaryngol Head Neck Surg. 2004;131(4):372–7.

Fletcher SM, Blair PA. Chronic halitosis from tonsilloliths: a common etiology. J La State Med Soc. 1988;140(6):7–9.

Karli R, Ak M, Karli A. A different placement of the stone; rhinolithiasis. Eur Rev Med Pharmacol Sci. 2012;16(11):1541–5.

Kato H, Yoshida A, Awano S, Ansai T, Takehara T. Quantitative detection of volatile sulfur compound-producing microorganisms in oral specimens using real-time PCR. Oral Dis. 2005;11(Suppl 1):67–71.

Katz HP, Katz JR, Bernstein M, Marcin J. Unusual presentation of nasal foreign bodies in children. JAMA. 1979;241(14):1496. https://doi.org/10.1001/jama.1979.03290400056026.

Kiger JR, Brenkert TE, Losek JD. Nasal foreign body removal in children. Pediatr Emerg Care. 2008;24(11):785–92 . quiz 790–2. https://doi.org/10.1097/PEC.0b013e31818c2cb9.

Kurul S, Kandogan T. Pharyngeal foreign body in a child persisting for three years. Emerg Med J. 2002;19(4):361–2. https://doi.org/10.1136/emj.19.4.361.

Leo G, Incorvaia C, Cazzavillan A, Consonni D. May chronic rhinosinusitis in children be diagnosed by clinical symptoms? Int J Pediatr Otorhinolaryngol.
2015;79(6):825–8. https://doi.org/10.1016/j.ijporl.2015.03.011.

Monteiro-Amado F, Chinellato LE, de Rezende ML. Evaluation of oral and nasal halitosis parameters in patients with repaired cleft lip and/or palate. Oral Surg Oral Med Oral Pathol Oral Radiol Endod. 2005;100(6):682–7. https://doi.org/10.1016/j.tripleo.2005.03.019.

Perera H, Fernando SM, Yasawardena AD, Karunaratne I. Prevalence of attention deficit hyperactivity disorder (ADHD) in children presenting with self-inserted nasal and aural foreign bodies. Int J Pediatr Otorhinolaryngol. 2009;73(10):1362–4. https://doi.org/10.1016/j.ijporl.2009.06.011.

Quirynen M, Dadamio J, Van den Velde S, De Smit M, Dekeyser C, Van Tornout M, Vandekerckhove B. Characteristics of 2000 patients who visited a halitosis clinic. J Clin Periodontol. 2009;36(11):970–5. https://doi.org/10.1111/j.1600-051X.2009.01478.x.

Rio AC, Franchi-Teixeira AR, Nicola EM. Relationship between the presence of tonsilloliths and halitosis in patients with chronic caseous tonsillitis. Br Dent J. 2008;204(2):E4. https://doi.org/10.1038/bdj.2007.1106.

Rosenberg M. Clinical assessment of bad breath: current concepts. J Am Dent Assoc. 1996;127(4):475–82.

Rosenberg M, Leib E. Experiences of an Israeli malodor clinic. In: Rosenberg M, editor. Bad breath research perspectives. Tel Aviv: Ramot Publishing—Tel Aviv University; 1997. p. 137–48.

Seemann R, Bizhang M, Djamchidi C, Kage A, Nachnani S. The proportion of pseudo-halitosis patients in a multidisciplinary breath malodour consultation. Int Dent J. 2006;56(2):77–81. https://doi.org/10.1111/j.1875-595X.2006.tb00077.x.

Stammberger H. Endoscopic endonasal surgery—concepts in treatment of recurring rhinosinusitis. Part I. Anatomic and pathophysiologic considerations. Otolaryngol Head Neck Surg. 1986;94(2):143–7. https://doi.org/10.1177/019459988609400202.

Syfert DF. Nasal foreign bodies and bromidrosis. JAMA. 1979;242(10):1031. https://doi.org/10.1001/jama.1979.03300100013005.

Talebian A, Tazhibi M, Iranpoor R, Semyari H, Taherzadeh M. Relationship between tonsil odor and oral malodor: a clinical study on 48 Iranian patients. J Breath Res. 2008;2(017016):3pp.

Tatli MM, San I, Karaoglanoglu M. Paranasal sinus computed tomographic findings of children with chronic cough. Int J Pediatr Otorhinolaryngol. 2001;60(3):213–7. https://doi.org/10.1016/S0165-5876(01)00535-3.

Tsuneishi M, Yamamoto T, Kokeguchi S, Tamaki N, Fukui K, Watanabe T. Composition of the bacterial flora in tonsilloliths. Microbes Infect. 2006;8(9–10):2384–9.

Wong FW, King NM. The oral health of children with clefts—a review. Cleft Palate Craniofac J. 1998;35(3):248–54.

Breath Odors and the Gastrointestinal Tract

6

Contents

In the absence of well-informed science, people intuitively associate breath odors with the digestive system. Perhaps, the stomach odors that arise transiently during eructation (burping) lead many to assume that breath odor may originate in the stomach. Old medical texts on this topic (Howe 1898; Shifman et al. 2002) cite indigestion, constipation, and dyspepsia as potential causes of breath odors further illustrates this point. Even nowadays, patients complaining of breath odors to their physicians or dentists are sometimes referred to the gastroenterologist (Delanghe et al. 1996).

Most researchers agree that the gastrointestinal tract is rarely involved in breath odor production. The esophagus is a closed flat tube, and odors are unlikely to be steadily released into the oral cavity. Yet, some other investigators have provided evidence support a possible link between breath odor and various gastrointestinal diseases and symptoms. At first these were mostly anecdotal observations such as case reports linking between pyloric stenosis and halitosis (Tydd and Dyer 1974). However, large controlled studies also showed higher prevalence of halitosis in patients suffering from inflammatory

bowel diseases (Katz et al. 2003). Most of these studies focused on two gastrointestinal conditions; reflux and *Helicobacter pylori* infection.

6.1 Gastroesophageal Reflux Disease (GERD)

Reflux (regurgitation) commonly referred to as heartburn is the emersion of the acidic content of the stomach back up into the esophagus. Although no rationale has been offered as to why this specific condition was considered as a cause for breath odors, several studies (Di Fede et al. 2008; Moshkowitz et al. 2007; Struch et al. 2008) reported a possible association between GERD and halitosis (Table 6.1). However, rather than relying on objective parameters (e.g., odor judge, sulfide levels), these studies based their diagnosis on self-reported breath odor questionnaires. Unfortunately, when it comes to halitosis, self-perception is notably unreliable (for further details, see Chap. 10). Furthermore, the largest of these studies (Struch et al. 2008) conducted in a general population (over 3000 participants)

© Springer Nature Switzerland AG 2020
N. Sterer, M. Rosenberg, *Breath Odors*, https://doi.org/10.1007/978-3-030-44731-1_6

Table 6.1 Reflux and halitosis

References	Aims	Malodor criteria	Findings	Criticism and comments
Carr et al. (2000)	ENT symptoms and gastroesophageal reflux disease (GERD) in small children ($n = 295$)	Charts review	15% halitosis in GERD+ 24% halitosis in GERD−	
Moshkowitz et al. (2007)	Possible association bet GERD and halitosis ($n = 132$)	Questionnaire	Halitosis was associated with GERD, heartburn, belching, and sour taste	Self-reported
Struch et al. (2008)	Self-reported halitosis and GERD in general population ($n = 3005$)	Interview: "do you often suffer from bad taste in your mouth or from bad breath?"	GERD-related symptoms (heartburn, acid regurgitation) were associated with halitosis subjects complaining of halitosis had more gingival bleeding and PPD > 4 mm	Self-reported (+associating bad taste with bad breath)
Di Fede et al. (2008)	Oral manifestations in GERD ($n = 400$)	"Subjective halitosis"	49% halitosis in GERD+ 31% halitosis in GERD− ($p = 0.0004$)	Self-reported
Kislig et al. (2013)	Halitosis in erosive and no-erosive GERD ($n = 66$)	Odor judge Halimeter Questionnaire	No association between halitosis and GERD-related erosions	
Lee et al. (2014)	Association between halitosis and GERD ($n = 54$)	Halimeter Questionnaire	No association between halitosis and GERD	

considered both "bad breath" and "bad taste in your mouth" as positive for halitosis. Another criticism is that oral conditions, more commonly associated with breath odors, were not taken into account. For example, in the same study mentioned above, subjects self-reporting of halitosis had higher prevalence of gingival bleeding which is directly related to oral malodor.

Another study (Carr et al. 2000) conducted in small children with or without GERD by reviewing their medical charts did not show any difference between the prevalence of halitosis in GERD positive and controls. Two additional studies (Kislig et al. 2013; Lee et al. 2014) employing objective measurements of malodor (odor judge) and malodor-related parameters (sulfide monitor) have reported no association between reflux disease and breath odors.

6.2 Helicobacter pylori (Hp) Infection

H. pylori (*Hp*) is a spiral Gram-negative bacterium that has been associated with gastritis, gastric ulcer, and cancer. Associating *Hp* with breath malodor started with an anecdotal observation. In the mid-1980s, Marshall ingested laboratory grown *Hp* in purpose of developing gastritis and fulfilling Koch's postulate (Marshall et al. 1985). While being infected, his colleagues noticed a "putrid" odor on his breath.

Several studies were conducted in order to test the possible association between *Hp* infection and breath odors (Table 6.2). Some of these studies (Gasbarrini et al. 1998; Moshkowitz et al. 2007; Schubert et al. 1992; Werdmuller et al. 2000) failed to find a link between the two. Again, these studies relied on self-reported halitosis rather than an objective means as the criterion for determining the presence of breath odors. Furthermore, few if any attempts were made to examine possible oral causes for the presence of malodor. Conversely, other studies (Candelli et al. 2003; Claus et al. 1996; Li et al. 2005) did show an association between *Hp* infection and halitosis. One of these (Claus et al. 1996) relied on objective parameters (i.e., odor judge scores and GC measurements) in order to establish the presence of halitosis. Moreover, oral malodor-related parameters (PI–plaque index, GI–gingival index, PPD–periodontal pockets depth,

Table 6.2   *Hp* and halitosis

References	Aims	Malodor/oral parameters	Findings and conclusions	Criticism and comments
Schubert et al. (1992)	Symptoms, gastritis and *Hp*	Interview *Hp*: biopsy	No correlation between *Hp* and halitosis	Self-reported
Gasbarrini et al. (1998)	*Hp* infection and GI symptoms in IDDM	*Hp*: [^{13}C] urea breath test	Prevalence of halitosis did not differ between *Hp*+ and *Hp*− groups	Self-reported
Werdmuller et al. (2000)	Clinical presentation of functional dyspepsia in *Hp*+ (*n* = 222) and Hp− (*n* = 182) pat.	Halitosis by questionnaire *Hp*: biopsy	*Hp*+ 29% halitosis *Hp*− 34% halitosis Conc: combination of retrosternal pain, weight loss, food intolerance and absence of halitosis were predictive for *Hp* infection	Self-reported
Moshkowitz et al. (2007)	GERD and halitosis	Questionnaire *Hp*: rapid urease test (CLO test)	No correlation was found between Hp infection status and halitosis occurrence and severity	Self-reported
Claus et al. (1996)	Halitosis and *Hp* (*n* = 80; 31*Hp*+, 49*Hp*−)	OJ GC *Hp*: [^{13}C] urea breath test	Significantly higher mouth air malodor and H$_2$S levels in *Hp*+ No difference in oral health parameters (PI, GI, PPD, TC)	44.7 mean age for *Hp*+ 33.8 mean age for *Hp*−
Candelli et al. (2003)	*Hp* and GI symptoms in IDDM	Questionnaire *Hp*: [^{13}C] urea breath test	Higher prevalence of halitosis in *Hp*+ then *Hp*− and in diabetics then controls	However, after correction for age, the difference was not significant. Self-reported
Li et al. (2005)	Dyspeptic symptoms (*n* = 782)	Questionnaire	Halitosis was more often found in dyspeptic patients with *Hp* infection ($p < 0.01$)	Self-reported
Tangerman et al. (2012)	Halitosis and *Hp* (*n* = 49; 11*Hp*+, 38*Hp*−)	OJ GC *Hp*: biopsy	No association between halitosis and *Hp* infection	

TC–tongue coating) were also determined. Results of this study showed significantly higher mouth air malodor and H$_2$S levels in *Hp*-positive subjects, whereas no difference was seen in oral health parameters (however, they did differ in age groups). Interestingly, this study links between the presence of an *Hp* infection and breath odors of oral origin (mouth air) rather than extra oral origin (lung air). However, a further study employing objective malodor measurements (odor judge and gas chromatography) found no association between breath odors and *Hp* infection (Tangerman et al. 2012).

Another factor that may cause physicians to link *Hp* infection and breath odors is the clinical observation that the malodor tends to disappear following *Hp* eradication treatment (Table 6.3). The first report to this effect was published in the early 1990s (Tiomny et al. 1992) showing the disappearance of breath malodor (as reported by respective family members) in four out of five patients following *Hp* eradication treatment (4 weeks) with metronidazole (although an earlier case report by Tydd in 1974 showed the same effect with tetracycline in pyloric stenosis patients). Several other larger studies (Ierardi et al. 1998; Katsinelos et al. 2007; Serin et al. 2003; Shashidhar et al. 2000) have reported similar results. However, malodor production is for the most part bacterial in origin and any use of antibiotics, especially those targeted against Gram-negatives and anaerobes such as metronidazole would be expected to affect the oral population of malodor-producing bacteria and decrease or eliminate the malodor for a certain period of time.

To shed more light on this problem, one study (Ierardi et al. 1998) employed an antiseptic

Table 6.3 *Hp* eradication therapy and halitosis

References	Aims	Malodor/*Hp* criteria (intervention)	Findings and conclusions	Criticism and comments
Tiomny et al. (1992)	Halitosis and *Hp* In three couples in which one or both had halitosis	Halitosis: Reported by a family member *Hp*: Biopsy [^{14}C] urea breath test (metronidazole)	Halitosis disappeared following treatment (4 weeks)	
Ierardi et al. (1998)	Halitosis and *Hp* in dyspeptic pat. complaining of halitosis 52/58(90%) had objective halitosis: 30(57%) *Hp*+22(43%)*Hp*−	Halitosis: Halimeter >190 ppb *Hp*: [^{13}C] urea breath test (amoxicillin/CHX mw/metronidazole)	In *Hp* persistent (11/30) CHX mw showed no effect on VSC but following metronidazole use in 9/11 *Hp* and halitosis disappeared	"Sulfide levels decreased without declining to below the cut off value even in the patients whose eradication treatment was unsuccessful"
Shashidhar et al. (2000)	*Hp* eradication in children (*n* = 28; 11 years)	Halitosis: questionnaire (patient + parent) *Hp*: biopsy (clarithromycin, amoxicillin)	Eradication achieved in 56% Halitosis before reported in 45% after in 22%	No significant correlation was observed between level of infection and pretreatment symptoms
Serin et al. (2003)	Halitosis as an indication for *Hp* eradication therapy (*n* = 148)	Halitosis: questionnaire (patient + relatives) *Hp*: biopsy (clarithromycin, amoxicillin) 4–6 weeks follow-up	Halitosis was resolved regardless of eradication status, but more significantly in the eradicated group	After the follow-up period halitosis was not reevaluated
Katsinelos et al. (2007)	Eradication therapy *Hp* halitosis: long-term outcome (*n* = 18)	Halitosis: questionnaire (patient + relatives) *Hp*: [^{13}C] urea breath test (clarithromycin, amoxicillin/ metronidazole, tetracycline)	Halitosis was resolved in 16/18 (over 6–108 months follow-up)	

mouthwash-containing chlorhexidine as a control showing no effect on oral volatile sulfide compounds levels in *Hp*+ subjects, whereas eradication therapy did reduce them. Another study (Katsinelos et al. 2007) offered long-term follow-up that showed the resolving of the malodor over a period of more than 6 months.

Nevertheless, other reports (Delanghe et al. 1996) and clinical experience shows that 3–6 weeks following the end of the antibiotic course, the malodor gradually returns even though *Hp* was completely eradicated from the stomach.

Although some studies imply an association between *Hp* infection and halitosis (Table 6.4), no satisfactory explanation has been offered as to how the two might be linked together. Several studies were carried out to investigate the pres-

ence of *Hp* in the oral cavity and its relation to oral malodor (Adler et al. 2005; Suzuki et al. 2008). One of these studies (Suzuki et al. 2008) found that subjects who were positive for *Hp* in their saliva had significantly more periodontal pockets and were also positive to periopathogenic bacteria (*Porphyromonas gingivalis, Treponema denticola, Prevotella intermedia*) all of which are known malodor producers. Although *Hp* has been shown to be able to produce volatile sulfide compounds on its own (Lee et al. 2006), a possible association with other VSC-producing bacteria which are much more abundant in the oral cavity might seem more reasonable.

In summary, most researchers agree that breath odor from the stomach is rare. Systemic antibiotics used to treat stomach ailments also suppress the oral microbiota, resulting in a tran-

Table 6.4 Oral *Hp* and halitosis

References	Aims/criteria	Malodor/oral parameters (intervention)	Findings and conclusions	Criticism and comments
Adler et al. (2005)	Oral *Hp* (PCR) associated with glossitis and halitosis	Halimeter >100 ppb	*Hp* was found in 87% of tongue biopsies of patients with glossitis and halitosis (but not in plaque and saliva) as compared to 2.6% in the control	
Suzuki et al. (2008)	Salivary *Hp* (PCR) and halitosis	OJ 0–5, GC PPD ≥5 mm TC 0–4 Saliva flow PCR periopathogens: Pg, Td, Pi	No difference between *Hp*+ and *Hp*− in malodor, total VSC and TC, but significantly higher PPD, methyl mercaptan, and periopathogens	

sient reduction in malodor that is sometimes erroneously interpreted as odor from the stomach. Several isolated studies show positive correlations comparing *Hp* and breath odor; these warrant further study.

References

Adler I, Denninghoff VC, Alvarez MI, Avagnina A, Yoshida R, Elsner B. Helicobacter pylori associated with glossitis and halitosis. Helicobacter. 2005;10(4):312–7.

Candelli M, Rigante D, Marietti G, Nista EC, Crea F, Bartolozzi F, Schiavino A, Pignataro G, Silveri NG, Gasbarrini G, Gasbarrini A. Helicobacter pylori, gastrointestinal symptoms, and metabolic control in young type 1 diabetes mellitus patients. Pediatrics. 2003;111(4 Pt 1):800–3.

Carr MM, Nguyen A, Nagy M, Poje C, Pizzuto M, Brodsky L. Clinical presentation as a guide to the identification of GERD in children. Int J Pediatr Otorhinolaryngol. 2000;54(1):27–32.

Claus D, Geypens B, Rutgeerts P, Ghyselen J, Hoshi K, Van Steenberghe D, Ghoos Y. Where gastroenterology and periodontology meets: determination of oral volatile organic compounds using closed loop trapping and high resolution gas chromatography ion trap detection. In: Van Steenberghe D, Rosenberg M, editors. Bad breath a multidisciplinary approach. Leuven: Leuven University Press; 1996. p. 15–27.

Delanghe G, Ghyselen J, Feenstra L, Van Steenberghe D. Experiences of a Belgian multidisciplinary breath odour clinic. In: Van Steenberghe D, Rosenberg M, editors. Bad breath a multy disciplinary approach. Leuven: Leuven University Press; 1996. p. 199–208.

Di Fede O, Di Liberto C, Occhipinti G, Vigneri S, Lo Russo L, Fedele S, Lo Muzio L, Campisi G. Oral manifestations in patients with gastro-oesophageal reflux disease: a single-center case-control study. J Oral Pathol Med. 2008;37(6):336–40.

Gasbarrini A, Ojetti V, Pitocco D, De Luca A, Franceschi F, Candelli M, Sanz Torre E, Pola P, Ghirlanda G, Gasbarrini G. Helicobacter pylori infection in patients affected by insulin-dependent diabetes mellitus. Eur J Gastroenterol Hepatol. 1998;10(6):469–72.

Howe JW. The breath, and the diseases which give it a fetid odor. 4th ed. New York: D. Appleton and Company; 1898.

Ierardi E, Amoruso A, La Notte T, Francavilla R, Castellaneta S, Marrazza E, Monno RA, Francavilla A. Halitosis and helicobacter pylori: a possible relationship. Dig Dis Sci. 1998;43(12):2733–7.

Katsinelos P, Tziomalos K, Chatzimavroudis G, Vasiliadis T, Katsinelos T, Pilpilidis I, Triantafillidis I, Paroutoglou G, Papaziogas B. Eradication therapy in helicobacter pylori-positive patients with halitosis: long-term outcome. Med Princ Pract. 2007;16(2):119–23.

Katz J, Shenkman A, Stavropoulos F, Melzer E. Oral signs and symptoms in relation to disease activity and site of involvement in patients with inflammatory bowel disease. Oral Dis. 2003;9(1):34–40.

Kislig K, Wilder-Smith CH, Bornstein MM, Lussi A, Seemann R. Halitosis and tongue coating in patients with erosive gastroesophageal reflux disease versus nonerosive gastroesophageal reflux disease. Clin Oral Investig. 2013;17(1):159–65.

Lee H, Kho HS, Chung JW, Chung SC, Kim YK. Volatile sulfur compounds produced by helicobacter pylori. J Clin Gastroenterol. 2006;40(5):421–6.

Lee HJ, Kim HM, Kim N, Oh JC, Jo HJ, Lee JT, Chang HY, Chang NH, Ahn S, Lee JY. Association between halitosis diagnosed by a questionnaire and halimeter and symptoms of gastroesophageal reflux disease. J Neurogastroenterol Motil. 2014;20(4):483–90.

Li XB, Liu WZ, Ge ZZ, Zhang DR, Zhao YJ, Dai J, Xue HB, Xiao SD. Analysis of clinical characteristics of dyspeptic symptoms in Shanghai patients. Chin J Dig Dis. 2005;6(2):62–7.

Marshall BJ, Armstrong JA, McGechie DB, Glancy RJ. Attempt to fulfil Koch's postulates for pyloric campylobacter. Med J Aust. 1985;142(8):436–9.

Moshkowitz M, Horowitz N, Leshno M, Halpern Z. Halitosis and gastroesophageal reflux disease: a possible association. Oral Dis. 2007;13(6):581–5.

Schubert TT, Schubert AB, Ma CK. Symptoms, gastritis, and helicobacter pylori in patients referred for endoscopy. Gastrointest Endosc. 1992;38(3):357–60.

Serin E, Gumurdulu Y, Kayaselcuk F, Ozer B, Yilmaz U, Boyacioglu S. Halitosis in patients with helicobacter pylori-positive non-ulcer dyspepsia: an indication for eradication therapy? Eur J Intern Med. 2003;14(1):45–8.

Shashidhar H, Peters J, Lin CH, Rabah R, Thomas R, Tolia V. A prospective trial of lansoprazole triple therapy for pediatric helicobacter pylori infection. J Pediatr Gastroenterol Nutr. 2000;30(3):276–82.

Shifman A, Orenbuch S, Rosenberg M. Bad breath—a major disability according to the Talmud. Isr Med Assoc J. 2002;4(10):843–5.

Struch F, Schwahn C, Wallaschofski H, Grabe HJ, Volzke H, Lerch MM, Meisel P, Kocher T. Self-reported halitosis and gastro-esophageal reflux disease in the general population. J Gen Intern Med. 2008;23(3):260–6.

Suzuki N, Yoneda M, Naito T, Iwamoto T, Masuo Y, Yamada K, Hisama K, Okada I, Hirofuji T. Detection of helicobacter pylori DNA in the saliva of patients complaining of halitosis. J Med Microbiol. 2008;57(Pt 12):1553–9.

Tangerman A, Winkel EG, de Laat L, van Oijen AH, de Boer WA. Halitosis and helicobacter pylori infection. J Breath Res. 2012;6(1):017102.

Tiomny E, Arber N, Moshkowitz M, Peled Y, Gilat T. Halitosis and helicobacter pylori. A possible link? J Clin Gastroenterol. 1992;15(3):236–7.

Tydd TF, Dyer NH. Pyloric stenosis presenting with halitosis. Br Med J. 1974;3(5926):321.

Werdmuller BF, van der Putten TB, Balk TG, Lamers CB, Loffeld RJ. Clinical presentation of helicobacter pylori-positive and -negative functional dyspepsia. J Gastroenterol Hepatol. 2000;15(5):498–502.

Other Sources of Breath Odors

Content

Although relatively rare, especially among the ambulatory population, breath odors may be a sign of a systemic condition or a metabolic disorder (Table 7.1). Usually, this symptom will appear in a later stage of the disease when the patient is already diagnosed. However, sometimes the breath odor may be an early sign or even the only sign for the underlying disorder or disease.

More commonly, exogenous sources such as food substances, smoking, or medications may also play a part in breath odor formation (Table 7.1). These various sources may contribute odor components either directly from the upper respiratory tract or indirectly through the blood via alveolar air. The latter is also referred to as "blood borne halitosis" (Tangerman and Winkel 2010). In this case, the odor component is absorbed through the blood stream and released through the alveoli into the lung air. As such these breath odors would be expected to be present in both oral and nasal exhalations.

Breath odors may originate from neoplasm and infections of the lower respiratory tract such as bronchogenic carcinoma, bronchiectasis, and anaerobic pulmonary infection (Gordon et al. 1985; Lorber 1975; Preti et al. 1988). The chemical analysis of breath samples from patients with lung cancer has shown elevated levels of acetone, methylethylketone, and n-propanol (Gordon et al. 1985). Alternatively, putrid smell might appear following a secondary bacterial infection of the tumor. Although putrid breath odor typically appears relatively late in the course of an anaerobic lung infection, following other symptoms such as fever, cough, and chest pains, it has been reported that in some cases it can serve as an early sign of the disease (Lorber 1975).

The "odor of decaying apples" on the breath of patients with uncontrolled diabetes mellitus was first recorded in the late eighteenth century (Crofford et al. 1977). In uncontrolled patients this disease, which is termed "hunger in the midst of plenty," causes an increase in lipid metabolism that results in the ketonic breath. This results from the formation of acetone, acetoacetate, and β-hydroxybutyrate that are transferred from the blood to the alveolar air and exhaled through the breath (Rooth and Ostenson 1966). Furthermore, diabetes also affects oral health and may aggravate oral diseases and conditions (e.g., gingivitis, periodontitis, and decrease in saliva flow) that contribute to oral malodor production (Ship 2003).

Liver cirrhosis may give rise to a characteristic breath odor known as *Fetor hepaticus*. This is

Table 7.1 Some of the systemic and external sources of breath odors

Source	Odor characteristics	Odor components	References
Lung disease; Pulmonary infection, Lung cancer	Putrid	Acetone, methylethylketone, *n*-propanol	Lorber (1975) Gordon et al. (1985)
Diabetes mellitus (uncontrolled)	Fruity	Acetone, ketones	Rooth and Ostenson (1966)
Liver (hepatic) cirrhosis	Musty, fresh cadaver ("fetor hepaticus")	Dimethyl sulfide, ketones	Van den Velde et al. (2008)
Kidney (renal) failure, uremia	Ammoniac, urine like	Ammonia, dimethylamine, trimethylamine	Simenhoff et al. (1977)
Metabolic disorders; Trimethylaminuria (TMAU) Methanethiol oxidase (MTO) deficiency	Fish like ("fish odor syndrome") cabbage-like breath odor	Trimethylamine Methanethiol and dimethylsulfide	Preti et al. (1992) Pol et al. (2018)
Medication; Disulfiram Cysteamine	Sulfurous	Carbon disulfide Dimethyl sulfide	O'Reilly and Motley (1977) Besouw et al. (2007)
Food; Garlic Onion	Garlic Onion	Allyl methyl sulfide Methyl propyl—sulfide	Suarez et al. (1999)
Tobacco smoking; Cigars Cigarettes	"Smoker's breath"	Trimethyl pyridine dimethyl pyrazine	Bazemore et al. (2006)

a sweet, musty, or slightly fecal smell on the breath which sometimes resembles the smell of a fresh cadaver. The impaired liver function decreases the metabolism of various malodorous compounds such as dimethyl sulfide and other ketones causing their increased blood levels and appearance on the breath (Van den Velde et al. 2008).

"Uremic breath" is a typical breath odor of patients with end-stage chronic renal failure (CRF). This type of breath odor has been described as "ammoniacal," "urine-like," and "fetid" odor and was attributed mainly to amine compounds such as dimethylamine and trimethylamine (Simenhoff et al. 1977). As with liver cirrhosis and diabetes, this is also a blood-borne breath odor resulting from an organ failure and consequent elevated blood levels of the odorous compounds. However, in a study conducted on 50 CRF patients undergoing hemodialysis a significant reduction in VSCs levels was also reported following the procedure (Gulsahi et al. 2014).

Apart from organ failure (e.g., liver, kidneys, pancreas), an impaired metabolic pathway, typically resulting from inherited mutations of an enzyme coding gene, may also result in the accu-

mulation of an odorous metabolite in the blood. An example of such a metabolic disorder that forms another type of blood-borne breath odor is known as "fish odor syndrome" or TMAU (i.e., trimethylamineuria) (Leopold et al. 1990). This condition results from the impaired N-oxidation and secretion of trimethylamine, a choline metabolite, and is estimated to be present in various degrees in as high as 1% of the population (Ayesh et al. 1993). Another metabolic disorder recently reported to induce a cabbage-like breath odor is a mutation in the Selenium-binding protein 1 (SELENBP1) that was suggested by Pol and coworkers to function as a methanethiol oxidase (MTO). It was suggested that a deficiency in this enzyme's activity may result in extraoral halitosis induced by high levels of methanethiol and dimethylsulfide (Pol et al. 2018).

Various medications may also cause a type of blood-borne breath odors. For example, medications such as disulfiram and cysteamine have been previously shown to cause breath odors possibly through the formation of sulfurous compounds, mainly dimethyl sulfide (Besouw et al. 2007; Murata et al. 2003). Some researchers suggested that dimethyl sulfide is the only VSC molecule that is transportable by blood since –SH-containing

VSCs like hydrogen sulfide and methyl mercaptan quickly reacts with the blood by binding or oxidation (Tangerman and Winkel 2010). Since cysteamine shows better absorption through the small intestines an enteric-coated formulation was developed that showed a 50% reduction in the side effect of dimethyl sulfide production (Besouw et al. 2012).

Some food substances such as onion and garlic contains sulfurous compounds such as allyl methyl sulfide and methyl propyl sulfide that can cause distinctive breath odors lasting up to 72 h following ingestion (Suarez et al. 1999). Although most of the malodor emanates directly from remnants in the oral cavity, mid 1930s research showed a distinct blood-borne element to garlic breath by feeding the garlic straight into the stomach and detecting it on the breath after several hours (Blankenhorn and Richards 1936).

Another common external source for breath odor is tobacco smoke. Smoking habits often cause a characteristic "ashtray like smell" known as "smoker's breath." The chemical analysis of tobacco and tobacco smoke shows many volatile sulfide compounds (Stedman 1968). However, in a study conducted in the general population in Japan, no association was found between smoking habits and the oral levels of volatile sulfide compounds (Miyazaki et al. 1995). Another study on the chemical composition of cigars smoker's breath detected other odor components such as trimethyl pyridine and dimethyl pyrazine from various samples including tongue samples (Bazemore et al. 2006).

In summary, bad breath from systemic conditions is rare among the ambulatory population. When odors emanate from the lungs or bronchi, both oral and nasal exhalations should express them, both in terms of characteristic smell and intensity.

References

Ayesh R, Mitchell SC, Zhang A, Smith RL. The fish odour syndrome: biochemical, familial, and clinical aspects. BMJ. 1993;307(6905):655–7.

Bazemore R, Harrison C, Greenberg M. Identification of components responsible for the odor of cigar smoker's breath. J Agric Food Chem. 2006;54(2):497–501.

Besouw M, Blom H, Tangerman A, de Graaf-Hess A, Levtchenko E. The origin of halitosis in cystinotic patients due to cysteamine treatment. Mol Genet Metab. 2007;91(3):228–33.

Besouw M, Tangerman A, Cornelissen E, Rioux P, Levtchenko E. Halitosis in cystinosis patients after administration of immediate-release cysteamine bitartrate compared to delayed-release cysteamine bitartrate. Mol Genet Metab. 2012;107(1–2):234–6.

Blankenhorn MA, Richards CE. Garlic breath odor. J Am Med Assoc. 1936;107(6):409–10.

Crofford OB, Mallard RE, Winton RE, Rogers NL, Jackson JC, Keller U. Acetone in breath and blood. Trans Am Clin Climatol Assoc. 1977;88:128–39.

Gordon SM, Szidon JP, Krotoszynski BK, Gibbons RD, O'Neill HJ. Volatile organic compounds in exhaled air from patients with lung cancer. Clin Chem. 1985;31(8):1278–82.

Gulsahi A, Evirgen S, Öztaş B, Genç Y, Çetinel Y. Volatile sulphur compound levels and related factors in patients with chronic renal failure. J Clin Periodontol. 2014;41(8):814–9.

Leopold DA, Preti G, Mozell MM, Youngentob SL, Wright HN. Fish-odor syndrome presenting as dysosmia. Arch Otolaryngol Head Neck Surg. 1990;116(3):354–5.

Lorber B. "Bad breath": presenting manifestation of anaerobic pulmonary infection. Am Rev Respir Dis. 1975;112(6):875–7.

Miyazaki H, Sakao S, Katoh Y, Takehara T. Correlation between volatile sulfur compounds and certain oral health measurements in the general population. J Periodontol. 1995;66(8):679–84.

Murata T, Fujiyama Y, Yamaga T, Miyazaki H. Breath malodor in an asthmatic patient caused by side-effects of medication: a case report and review of the literature. Oral Dis. 2003;9(5):273–6.

O'Reilly RA, Motley CH. Breath odor after disulfiram. JAMA. 1977;238(24):2600.

Pol A, Renkema GH, Tangerman A, Winkel EG, Engelke UF, de Brouwer APM, Lloyd KC, Araiza RS, van den Heuvel L, Omran H, Olbrich H, Oude Elberink M, Gilissen C, Rodenburg RJ, Sass JO, Schwab KO, Schäfer H, Venselaar H, Sequeira JS, Op den Camp HJM, Wevers RA. Mutations in SELENBP1, encoding a novel human methanethiol oxidase, cause extraoral halitosis. Nat Genet. 2018;50(1):120–9.

Preti G, Labows JN, Kostelc JG, Aldinger S, Daniele R. Analysis of lung air from patients with bronchogenic carcinoma and controls using gas chromatography-mass spectrometry. J Chromatogr. 1988;432:1–11.

Preti G, Clark L, Cowart BJ, Feldman RS, Lowry LD, Weber E, Young IM. Non-oral etiologies of oral malodor and altered chemosensation. J Periodontol. 1992;63(9):790–6.

Rooth G, Ostenson S. Acetone in alveolar air, and the control of diabetes. Lancet. 1966;2(7473):1102–5.

Ship JA. Diabetes and oral health: an overview. J Am Dent Assoc. 2003;134(Spec No):4S–10S.

Simenhoff ML, Burke JF, Saukkonen JJ, Ordinario AT, Doty R. Biochemical profile or uremic breath. N Engl J Med. 1977;297(3):132–5.

Stedman RL. The chemical composition of tobacco and tobacco smoke. Chem Rev. 1968;68(2):153–207.

Suarez F, Springfield J, Furne J, Levitt M. Differentiation of mouth versus gut as site of origin of odoriferous breath gases after garlic ingestion. Am J Phys. 1999;276(2 Pt 1):G425–30.

Tangerman A, Winkel EG. Extra—oral halitosis: an overview. J Breath Res. 2010;4(017003):6pp.

Van den Velde S, Nevens F, Van Hee P, van Steenberghe D, Quirynen M. GC-MS analysis of breath odor compounds in liver patients. J Chromatogr B Analyt Technol Biomed Life Sci. 2008;875(2):344–8.

Measurements of Breath Odors and Related Parameters

8

Contents

Breath odors, much like other odor nuisances (e.g., sewage, garbage, livestock waste), are perceived in everyday life by our sense of smell. The human nose can pick up the scent of a large variety of different odorants at very low concentrations that are sometimes below instrumental detection thresholds. That is why organoleptic measurements employing human odor judges are still considered the "golden standard" in various odor-testing scenarios, including breath odors evaluation both for research and the clinical setting.

However, organoleptic measurement by a human odor judge has a few drawbacks, including potential lack of objectivity and interpersonal variation. To overcome this, a panel of judges is often employed and training methods are carried out. Adjunct instrumental methods for measuring malodor-related parameters have been devised, including the instrumental measurement of volatile sulfides and other malodor-associated components, as well as microbial and biochemical assays.

8.1 Odor Judge Scoring

Environmental odor nuisances are generally judged by various criteria collectively known as the FIDO factors (Mackie et al. 1998). These

© Springer Nature Switzerland AG 2020
N. Sterer, M. Rosenberg, *Breath Odors*, https://doi.org/10.1007/978-3-030-44731-1_8

include frequency (number of odor occurrences in a given time), intensity (strength of odor), duration (period of time for odor occurrence), and offensiveness (unpleasantness or character of odor). However, in the case of breath odors, odor intensity scales are considered the main tool for odor quantification both for research and clinical proposes. On some occasions (e.g., breath fresheners testing) hedonic scales measuring offensiveness/pleasantness characteristics may also be employed.

Due to the importance attributed to odor intensity in the determination of an odor problem, various odor intensity rating methods have been developed. These can be divided into two categories: scaling and dilution. Scaling involves grading the intensity of the malodor using a scale ranging from "no odor" to "extremely strong odor" either dichotomously (present or absent) or with intermittent-level criteria (e.g., "faint," "moderate" ext.) on a typical 4-, 5-, or 6-point scale. Dilution methods are based on mixing the sample with odor free air in various concentrations in order to determine detectability or odor threshold concentration.

The most widely used odor intensity organoleptic scale in breath odor research is a 6-point scale (Table 8.1) also known as the "0–5 scale," and sometimes erroneously referred to as the "Rosenberg scale" (Rosenberg and McCulloch 1992), since it was first introduced by Allison and Katz (1919).

Generally, the odor judge or panelist evaluates the odor by directly or indirectly sniffing the exhaled mouth air at a fixed distance (e.g., 10 cm) from the subject's mouth, and scoring the odor according to the scale (Fig. 8.1). This can be done directly from the subject's mouth, or indirectly

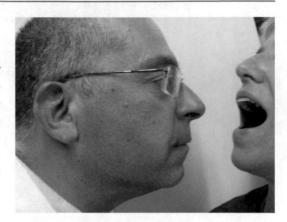

Fig. 8.1 Organoleptic (odor judge) assessment of breath odor

using a sampling bag. A partition screen has sometimes been applied to blind the odor judge to the subject's appearance (Murata et al. 2002). In some instances, the subject is asked to speak ("count to 20 test") thus allowing the odor judge to ascertain the odor level in a more natural manner.

In our initial studies, we adopted the "forced choice" approach, i.e., the judge was forced to choose one of the individual six categories (Rosenberg et al. 1991a). We continually faced the following dilemma. How does one score the level of an odor that is somewhere between slight and moderate? One possibility was to use a visual analogue continuous scale that is often used in other perception studies, e.g., to register the level of pain. Another approach is to allow judges to score in between the fixed points (e.g., give a score of 2.5, between slight and moderate) (Greenstein et al. 1997). When the sample size is large (e.g. $n = 100$), the results approximate data obtained using a continuous scale (Goldberg et al. 1994). Statistical tools developed for analyzing continuous data (e.g., linear regression analysis, Pearson correlation coefficients) can then be employed with greater confidence.

Interpersonal variation in odor perception between judges remains a major problem (Rosenberg et al. 1991b). In order to try and standardize odor judge scoring, calibration and training methods have been proposed. Odor judge

Table 8.1 Breath odor intensity scale (organoleptic scale)

Odor intensity level	Level description
0	No odor
1	Barley noticeable odor
2	Slight but clearly noticeable odor
3	Moderate odor
4	Strong odor
5	Extremely strong odor

training protocol based on the American Society of Testing and Materials Standards (introduction to sensory scales, use of *n*-butanol reference and sniffing techniques) was shown to reduce odor judge errors (Nachnani et al. 2005).

Dilution methods are usually device dependent. They are based on an apparatus or instrument designed to mix and dilute the odor sample to a set of concentrations enabling the judge to determine the minimal odor detectability or odor threshold. Some of these devices are handheld and used in field studies (e.g., olfactometer). In early studies on oral malodor done by Fosdick and colleagues they reported the use of a device called the osmoscope as a sample dilution method designed to determine odor intensity (Brening et al. 1939).

Recently, a non-apparatus-dependent dilution method was reported (Bornstein et al. 2009). This method relies on the distance between the odor judge's nose and the patient's mouth as the diluting factor (i.e., 1 m, 30 and 10 cm) assuming that a higher intensity malodor would be sensed from a greater distance. Whereas, organoleptic scales (continuous as possible) are more robust for research this simple method was deemed suitable for a clinical setting.

8.2   Instrumental Measuring of Malodor-Related Compounds

8.2.1   Gas Chromatography (GC)

The need for objective, quantitative techniques to serve as adjunct tests for the organoleptic measurement for both research and the clinic led to the development of various instrumental measuring techniques.

The use of gas chromatography for the quantification of volatile sulfide compounds (VSC) in mouth air was first reported by Tonzetich in the early 1970s (Tonzetich 1971). Since then many studies have employed this method and reported significant correlations between GC measurements of VSC and malodor levels as evaluated organoleptically by odor judges (Table 8.2).

Table 8.2 Association between gas chromatography measurement of mouth air VSC levels and oral malodor scores

References	Parameters	correlations
Schmidt et al. (1978) ($n = 102$)	Odor judge scores (0–3; 3 judges)	*Kendall correlation*
	Study I ($n = 36$)	$r = 0.28, p < 0.05$
	Study II ($n = 66$)	$r = 0.35, p < 0.001$
Shimura et al. (1996) ($n = 21$)		*Pearson correlation*
	Odor judge scores (0–4; 3 judges)	$r = 0.71, p < 0.01$
Oho et al. (2001) ($n = 155$)		*Spearman correlation*
	Odor judge scores (0–3; 3 judges)	$r = 0.69, p < 0.0001$
Amano et al. (2002) ($n = 61$)		*Spearman correlation*
	Odor judge scores (0–3; 3 judges)	$r = 0.47, p < 0.01$
Tanaka et al. (2004b) ($n = 78$)		*Spearman correlation*
	Odor judge scores (0–5; 1 judge)	$r = 0.63, p < 0.05$
Awano et al. (2004) ($n = 127$)	Odor judge scores (0–5; 3 judges)	*Spearman correlation*
	CH_3SH	$r = 0.75, p < 0.001$
	H_2S	$r = 0.59, p < 0.001$
	Total VSC	$r = 0.74, p < 0.001$
Nonaka et al. (2005) ($n = 66$)		*Correlation (not specified)*
	Odor judge scores (not specified)	$r = 0.73$, *p*- not specified
Hunter et al. (2005) ($n = 25$)	Odor judge scores (0–5; 2 judges)	*Pearson correlation*
	CH_3SH	$r = 0.61, p < 0.001$
	H_2S	$r = 0.63, p < 0.001$
	Total VSC	$r = 0.65, p < 0.001$

Traditional GC has a few distinctive disadvantages such as being time-consuming, costly, and requiring a professional technician for operation; conversely, it allows for the detection and quantitation of specific compounds. This feature has helped in the identification of various compounds present in mouth air and breath samples (see Chap. 3) and may help to identify the role of specific volatiles in malodor of various origins. For example, whereas hydrogen sulfide is produced largely from the tongue dorsum, methyl mercaptan is elevated in cases with periodontitis (Yaegaki and Sanada 1992). Furthermore, other non-sulfide compounds detected by GC (e.g., pyridine, picoline) were also associated with the presence of periodontal disease (Kostelc et al. 1981).

The technical complexity of GC along with the other drawbacks had limited its application mainly to research and rendered it unsuitable for the clinic. However, a simpler GC instrument suitable for clinical measurement has been recently introduced (Oralchroma®; Murata et al. 2006).

8.2.2 Sulfide Monitor

In the early 1990s, Rosenberg and coworkers suggested the use of a portable sulfide monitor, originally designed for ambient air quality measurement in working and living environments (Fig. 8.2) for the measurement of sulfide levels in mouth air (Rosenberg et al. 1991a, b). Although this device measures the total concentration of volatile sulfide compounds and does not distinguish between the individual sulfide compounds, its readings correlated significantly with odor judge scores in numerous studies (Table 8.3).

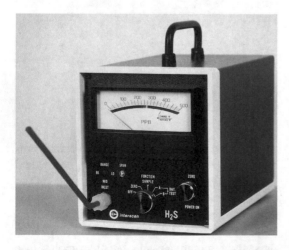

Fig. 8.2 Sulfide monitor (Interscan corp. CA) 1170 series

Table 8.3 Association between sulfide monitor (Halimeter®) measurement of mouth air VSC levels and oral malodor scores

References	Parameters	Correlations
Rosenberg et al. (1991b) (n = 75)		*Spearman correlation*
	Odor judge scores (0–5; 7 judges)	r = 0.60, p < 0.001
Rosenberg et al. (1991a) (n = 41)	Odor judge scores (0–5; 2 judges)	*Pearson correlation*
	Odor judge 1	r = 0.55, p < 0.0001
	Odor judge 2	r = 0.43, p < 0.0001
De Boever et al. (1994) (n = 55)		*Pearson correlation*
	Odor judge scores (0–4; 1 judge)	r = 0.63, p < 0.001
Kozlovsky et al. (1994) (n = 52)		*Pearson correlation*
	Odor judge scores (10 cm continuous scale; 1 judge)	r = 0.47, p < 0.001
Greenstein et al. (1997) (n = 123)	Odor judge scores (0–5; 2 judges)	*Pearson correlation*
	Odor judge 1	r = 0.27, p = 0.003
	Odor judge 2	r = 0.39, p < 0.001
Willis et al. (1999) (n = 30)		*Pearson correlation*
	Odor judge scores (0–10; 3 judges)	r = 0.41, p = 0.027
Oho et al. (2001) (n = 155)		*Spearman correlation*
	Odor judge scores (0–3; 3 judges)	r = 0.66, p < 0.0001
Sterer et al. (2002) (n = 64)	Odor judge scores (0–5; 2 judges)	*Spearman correlation*
	Odor judge 1	r = 0.37, p = 0.002
	Odor judge 2	r = 0.46, p < 0.001
Iwanicka-Grzegorek et al. (2005) (n = 124)		*Spearman correlation*
	Odor judge scores (0–5; 3 judges)	r = 0.78, p < 0.001
Stamou et al. (2005) (n = 71)		*Pearson correlation*
	Odor judge scores (0–5; 1 judge)	r = 0.59, p < 0.001
Sterer et al. (2008) (n = 42)		*Spearman correlation*
	Odor judge scores (0–5; 2 judges)	r = 0.66, p < 0.001

Table 8.3 (continued)

References	Parameters	Correlations
Vandekerckhove et al. (2009) (n = 280)	Odor judge scores (0–5; 1 judge)	*Spearman correlation* $r = 0.74$, $p < 0.01$
Dadamio et al. (2013) (n = 100)	Odor judge scores (0–5; 1 judge)	*Spearman correlation* $r = 0.63$, $p < 0.001$
Laleman et al. (2018) (n = 476)	Odor judge scores (0–5; 1 judge)	*Spearman correlation* $r = 0.48$, $p < 0.001$

Its simple operation, small size, rapid sample analysis, and relatively low cost made the sulfide monitor the most popular means for VSC measurements in both research and clinical settings. Furthermore, in studies carried out using both GC and sulfide monitor for measuring oral VSCs levels (Furne et al. 2002; Oho et al. 2001) the two correlated significantly with one another yielding correlation coefficients of 0.73 ($p < 0.01$) and 0.84 ($p < 0.0001$).

8.3 Measuring Techniques of Malodor-Related Compounds

Other measuring techniques for the detection of VSC as well as other malodor-related compounds (e.g., ammonia, amines) have been reported in the literature (Table 8.4). These include various methods ranging from simple colorimetric assays and small portable semiconductor based sulfide monitors to more complex approaches involving elaborate laboratory equipment such as chemical sensors array and high-performance liquid chromatography.

8.4 Biochemical Assays

8.4.1 BANA Test

In 1990, Loesche and coworkers (1990) suggested the use of the synthetic peptide benzoyl-DL-arginine-naphthylamide (BANA) as a diagnostic test for the presence of several anaerobic periopathogenic bacteria (i.e., *Treponema denticola*, *Porphyromonas gingivalis,* and *Bacteroides forsythus*). These bacteria possess a trypsin-like activity that enables them to break down a synthetic peptide attached to a color-producing indicator, yielding a color reaction indicative of their presence.

Since these bacteria are Gram-negative anaerobic bacteria that can produce malodorous compounds as a by-product of their proteolytic activity, it was suggested that the BANA test may serve as a diagnostic test for oral malodor and malodor-related microorganisms. Several studies have compared BANA test results from various oral samples (e.g., plaque, tongue coating, saliva) with odor judge scores and VSC levels (Table 8.5).

The data from these and other studies show that BANA testing of subgingival plaque samples especially from periodontal patients is more often associated with oral malodor as compared to saliva or tongue samples. However, the correlations, while significant, are lower than those obtained comparing odor judge scores and VSC levels.

8.4.2 β-Galactosidase Activity Assay

Some of the salivary proteins available for bacterial degradation are glycoproteins (e.g., salivary mucins) that are comprised of carbohydrate side chains surrounding a protein core. In order to expose the protein core and make it available for proteolytic degradation these side chains must first be removed. β-Galactosidase is a key enzyme in this deglycosylation process which is usually carried out by Gram-positive oral bacteria, mainly streptococci (Sterer and Rosenberg 2006).

In 2002, we reported that the activity of β-Galactosidase in saliva is associated with oral malodor scores (Sterer et al. 2002) suggesting that the quantification of the enzyme's activity in saliva may serve as a diagnostic tool for oral malodor (Fig. 8.3). Since then, further studies have been conducted to test this premise (Table 8.6).

Table 8.4 Association between malodor-related compounds measurement (chemical sensors, gas detectors, colorimetric assays, and chromatogray) and oral malodor scores

References	Compounds	Method	Correlations with malodor
Goldberg et al. (1994) ($n = 52$)	Cadaverine	High-performance liquid chromatography (HPLC)	Pearson correlation $r = 0.37, p = 0.027$
Shimura et al. (1997) ($n = 94$)	VSC	Portable monitor with a zinc-oxide thin-film semiconductor sensor	Pearson correlation $r = 0.82, p < 0.01$
Morita et al. (2001) ($n = 20$)	Sulfide ions	Sulfide electrode tongue probe	Spearman correlation $r = 0.77, p < 0.01$
Amano et al. (2002) ($n = 61$)	Ammonia	Portable ammonia-monitoring device	Pearson correlation $r = 0.16$, NS
Tanaka et al. (2004a) ($n = 78$)	Volatiles (low boiling point)	Chemical sensor array ("electronic nose")	Spearman correlation $r = 0.71, p < 0.05$
Iwanicka-Grzegorek et al. (2005) ($n = 124$)	Salivary amines (low molecular weight)	Ninhydrin method	Spearman correlation $r = 0.60, p < 0.001$
Sopapornamorn et al. (2006) ($n = 260$)	VSC	Portable monitor with a zinc-oxide thick-film semiconductor sensor	Pearson correlation $r = 0.64, p < 0.01$
Dadamio et al. (2011) ($n = 50$)	Salivary amines	Colorimetric assay	Spearman correlation $r = 0.49, p < 0.05$
Tamaki et al. (2011) ($n = 30$)	Reductive gases (e.g., VSC, ammonia)	Thin coat tin dioxide semiconductor gas sensor (BB checker)	Spearman correlation $r = 0.89, p < 0.001$
Dadamio et al. (2012) ($n = 100$)	Salivary amines	Colorimetric assay	Spearman correlation $r = 0.58, p < 0.01$
Dadamio et al. (2013) ($n = 100$)	VSC Reductive gases	GC (Oralchroma) GS (BB checker)	Spearman correlation $r = 0.68, p < 0.001$ $r = 0.13$, N.S.
Laleman et al. (2018) ($n = 476$)	VSC	GC (Oralchroma): H_2S CH_3SH $(CH_3)_2S$	Spearman correlation $r = 0.63, p < 0.001$ $r = 0.60, p < 0.001$ $r = 0.32, p < 0.001$

8.5   Cysteine Challenge

The addition of cysteine, a sulfur-containing amino acid, to incubated dental plaque (Tonzetich and Carpenter 1971), or a suspension of Gram-negative oral bacteria (Solis Gaffar et al. 1979), resulted in increased production of VSCs and malodor. Furthermore, when healthy subjects rinsed their mouths with a cysteine solution

(Wåler 1997) VSC production rose sharply especially from the tongue dorsum.

In 2002, Kleinberg (Kleinberg and Codipilly 2002) reported the use of a cysteine challenge testing based on successive rinsing with 5 mL of 6 mM cysteine solution for 30 s in 20 min intervals for a period of 7 h. Using these tests they demonstrated the effect of various oral cleansing procedures and products on VSC production in the mouth.

Table 8.5 Oral malodor parameters and the BANA test

References	Parameters/criteria		Findings
De Boever et al. (1994) ($n = 55$)	Malodor complaint	No complaint	Differences between groups (ANOVA)
	BANA tongue		NS[a]
	BANA plaque		$P < 0.05$
Kozlovsky et al. (1994) ($n = 52$)			*Spearman correlation*
	Odor judge[b] and BANA shallow pockets (<4 mm)		$r = 0.33, p = 0.016$
	Odor judge[b] and BANA deep pockets (≥4 mm)		$r = 0.26, p = 0.034$
	Odor judge[b] and BANA tongue		$r = 0.36, p = 0.008$
	Odor judge[b] and BANA saliva		$r = 0.36, p = 0.009$
Morita and Wang (2001) ($n = 81$)			*Pearson correlation*
	Odor judge[b] and BANA healthy sites(<4 mm)		$r = 0.02$, NS[a]
	Odor judge[b] and BANA low–moderate (4–6 mm)		$r = 0.27, p = 0.015$
	Odor judge[b] and BANA severe sites (>6 mm)		$r = 0.23, p = 0.042$
	Odor judge[b] and BANA tongue		$r = 0.27, p = 0.014$
Figueiredo et al. (2002) ($n = 41$)			*Pearson correlation*
	VSC[c] and BANA subgingival plaque (≤3 mm)		$r = 0.4$, NS[a]
	VSC[c] and BANA subgingival plaque (>3 mm)		$r = 0.55, p = 0.01$
	VSC[c] and BANA tongue		$r = 0.07–0.14$, NS[a]
	VSC[c] and BANA saliva		$r = 0.06–0.10$, NS[a]
Pham et al. (2012) ($n = 217$)	*Periodontitis group:*		*Pearson correlation*
	Odor judge[b] and BANA subgingival		$r = 0.74, p < 0.001$
	Odor judge[b] and BANA tongue		$r = 0.64, p < 0.001$
	Odor judge[b] and BANA saliva		$r = 0.35, p < 0.001$
	Gingivitis group:		
	Odor judge[b] and BANA subgingival		$r = 0.26, p = 0.018$
	Odor judge[b] and BANA tongue		$r = 0.62, p < 0.001$
	Odor judge[b] and BANA saliva		$r = 0.56, p < 0.001$

[a]*NS* nonsignificant
[b]Odor judge scores on a scale of 0–5
[c]Sulfide monitor (Halimeter) readings

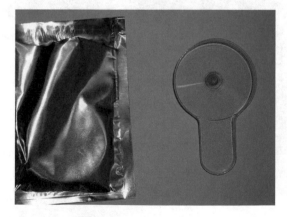

Fig. 8.3 β-galactosidase assay; color indicator (blue) correlates with malodor levels

8.6 Salivary Incubation Assays

Salivary incubation assays have been used over the past 60 years in oral malodor research. This system represents the complexity of the oral environment both in terms of bacterial diversity and substrate availability. Furthermore, this system tends to produce malodor components following brief anaerobic incubation of only a few hours.

Quirynen and coworkers (2003) reported the use of a salivary incubation assay in a pilot study of eight healthy subjects. Their results showed strong correlations between VSC measured from the saliva samples following 3 h anaerobic incubation and oral malodor scores as rated by an odor judge (Table 8.7). They concluded that salivary incubation assay may serve as an indirect method for oral malodor measurements.

Table 8.6 Oral malodor parameters and β-Galactosidase activity

Reference	Parameters		Findings
Sterer et al. (2002) (n = 64)			*Spearman correlation*
	Odor judge1[a] and β-Galactosidase assay		r = 0.38, p = 0.002
	Odor judge2[a] and β-Galactosidase assay		r = 0.47, p < 0.001
	VSC[b] and β-Galactosidase assay		r = 0.18, NS[c]
Stamou et al. (2005) (n = 71)			*Pearson correlation*
	Odor judge[a] and β-Galactosidase assay		r = 0.52, p = 0.001
	VSC[b] and β-Galactosidase assay		r = 0.38, p = 0.001
Rosenberg et al. (2007) (n = 88)			*Spearman correlation*
	Odor judge[a] and β-Galactosidase assay		r = 0.59, p < 0.001
	VSC[b] and β-Galactosidase assay		r = 0.31, p < 0.001
Yoneda et al. (2010) (n = 49)	β-Galactosidase positive (n = 10)	β-Galactosidase negative (n = 39)	Differences between groups (t-test)
	Odor judge[a]		p = 0.012
	VSC[b]		p < 0.001
Masuo et al. (2012) (n = 56)	*Periodontaly healthy group*: Odor judge[a]		*Pearson correlation* r = 0.4–0.7, p = 0.03
	VSC[d]		r = 0.66, p < 0.001
Petrini et al. (2012) (n = 94)			*Spearman correlation*
	Odor judge[a] and β-Galactosidase assay		r = 0.78, p < 0.001
Petrini et al. (2014) (n = 50)			*Spearman correlation*
	Odor judge[a] and β-Galactosidase assay		r = 0.64, p < 0.001

[a]Odor judge scores on a scale of 0–5
[b]Sulfide monitor (Halimeter) readings
[c]*NS* nonsignificant
[d]Gas chromatography (GC)

Table 8.7 Association between microbial assays and oral malodor parameters

References	Assay	Parameters	Association
Hartley et al. (1996) (n = 50)	Differential agar for H₂S-producing bacteria		*Regression analysis*
		Odor judge[a] and % black CFU[b]	r = 0.37, p < 0.001
Quirynen et al. (2003) (n = 8)	Salivary incubation assay		*Pearson correlation*
		Odor judge[c] and VSC[d] saliva[e]	r = 0.54, p < 0.001
Haraszthy et al. (2007) (n = 13)	Polymerase chain reaction (PCR)		χ^2 *analysis*
		Halitosis[a,d] and % S. moorei[f]	$\chi^2 = 0.22$, p < 0.05
Sterer et al. (2008) (n = 42)	Microscopic sulfide assay (MSA)		*Spearman correlation*
		Odor judge[a] and MSA scores[g]	r = 0.48, p = 0.001
Ueno et al. (2013) (n = 165)	Quantitative polymerase chain reaction (qPCR)		*Mann-Whitney (malodor vs non-malodor)*
		Odor judge[a] and total counts[h]	p = 0.02

[a]Odor judge scores (mouth air) on a scale of 0–5
[b]Black colonies on growth agar supplemented with ferrous sulfate
[c]Odor judge scores (mouth air) on a scale of 0–4
[d]Sulfide monitor (Halimeter) readings
[e]Following 3 h anaerobic incubation
[f]Identified by direct amplification of 16S ribosomal DNA
[g]Digital images analysis for black pixels (Image Pro Plus)
[h]From mouthrinse water

An attempt was made to find a salivary incubation assay that yields odor that more closely resembles breath odor (Goldberg et al. 1997). Among various additions, it was found that decarboxylase medium, when inoculated with saliva, produces an odor closely resembling the character of breath odor.

8.7 Microbial Assays

The identification of oral malodor-producing bacteria is based mainly on their ability to produce hydrogen sulfide. This is commonly done using a differential agar-containing lead or iron. These metal ions precipitate with the sulfide ions creating a black salt that stains the bacterial colony formed on the differential agar and allows for the enumeration of the putative malodor-producing bacteria in a given sample (Fig. 8.4). This method was used in order to show an association between oral malodor ratings and malodor-producing bacteria from tongue coating samples (Hartley et al. 1996); (Table 8.7).

However, this technique requires prolonged anaerobic incubation of up to 7 days. Further, it is limited to the detection of cultivable bacteria which comprise about 30% of the total bacterial population in the oral cavity. In 2008, we suggested a new technique based on the same principle but one that does not require bacterial

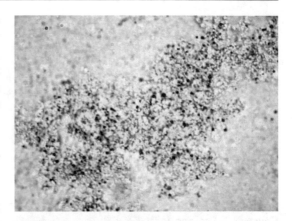

Fig. 8.5 Microscopic sulfide assay; VSC-producing bacteria are stained black (with permission from JBR)

cultivation (Sterer et al. 2008). We added the iron salt to samples of whole saliva that were kept overnight in 37 °C and the cell associated black precipitate was observed microscopically (Fig. 8.5). The black precipitate that was quantified by computerized analysis of the digital images captured from the microscopic slides was significantly associated with oral malodor levels in 42 subjects. ROC curve analysis showed the technique to have a diagnostic accuracy of 0.70 as compared to 0.78 for the Halimeter.

The study of cultivable and noncultivable bacteria using molecular techniques such as DNA hybridization and PCR have been used primarily for dichotomous comparisons of oral bacterial populations of halitosis-positive and negative patients (see Chap. 3). In some cases, associations between the PCR quantification of malodor associated bacteria and halitosis have also been demonstrated (Haraszthy et al. 2007).

References

Allison VC, Katz SH. An investigation of stenches and odors for industrial purposes. J Ind Eng Chem. 1919;11(4):336–8.

Amano A, Yoshida Y, Oho T, Koga T. Monitoring ammonia to assess halitosis. Oral Surg Oral Med Oral Pathol Oral Radiol Endod. 2002;94(6):692–6.

Awano S, Koshimune S, Kurihara E, Gohara K, Sakai A, Soh I, Hamasaki T, Ansai T, Takehara T. The assessment of methyl mercaptan, an important clinical marker for the diagnosis of oral malodor. J Dent. 2004;32(7):555–9.

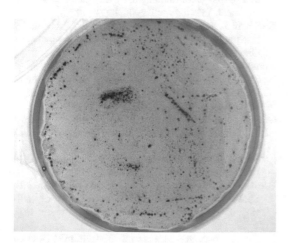

Fig. 8.4 Differentiating agar for VSC-producing bacteria (shown as black colonies)

Bornstein MM, Kislig K, Hoti BB, Seemann R, Lussi A. Prevalence of halitosis in the population of the city of Bern, Switzerland: a study comparing self-reported and clinical data. Eur J Oral Sci. 2009;117(3):261–7.

Brening RH, Sulser GF, Fosdick LS. The determination of halitosis by the use of the osmoscope and the cryoscopic method. J Dent Res. 1939;18(2):127–32.

Dadamio J, Van Tornout M, Van den Velde S, Federico R, Dekeyser C, Quirynen M. A novel and visual test for oral malodour: first observations. J Breath Res. 2011;5(4):046003.

Dadamio J, Van Tornout M, Vancauwenberghe F, Federico R, Dekeyser C, Quirynen M. Clinical utility of a novel colorimetric chair side test for oral malodour. J Clin Periodontol. 2012;39(7):645–50.

Dadamio J, Laleman I, De Geest S, Vancauwenberghe F, Dekeyser C, Coucke W, Quirynen M. Usefulness of a new malodour-compound detection portable device in oral malodour diagnosis. J Breath Res. 2013;7(4):046005.

De Boever EH, De Uzeda M, Loesche WJ. Relationship between volatile sulfur compounds, BANA-hydrolyzing bacteria and gingival health in patients with and without complaints of oral malodor. J Clin Dent. 1994;4(4):114–9.

Figueiredo LC, Rosetti EP, Marcantonio E Jr, Marcantonio RA, Salvador SL. The relationship of oral malodor in patients with or without periodontal disease. J Periodontol. 2002;73(11):1338–42.

Furne J, Majerus G, Lenton P, Springfield J, Levitt DG, Levitt MD. Comparison of volatile sulfur compound concentrations measured with a sulfide detector vs. gas chromatography. J Dent Res. 2002;81(2):140–3.

Goldberg S, Kozlovsky A, Gordon D, Gelernter I, Sintov A, Rosenberg M. Cadaverine as a putative component of oral malodor. J Dent Res. 1994;73(6):1168–72.

Goldberg S, Kozlovsky A, Rosenberg M. Association of diamines with oral malodor. In: Rosenberg M, editor. Bad breath research perspectives. Tel Aviv: Ramot Publishing Tel Aviv University; 1997. p. 71–85.

Greenstein RB, Goldberg S, Marku-Cohen S, Sterer N, Rosenberg M. Reduction of oral malodor by oxidizing lozenges. J Periodontol. 1997;68(12):1176–81.

Haraszthy VI, Zambon JJ, Sreenivasan PK, Zambon MM, Gerber D, Rego R, Parker C. Identification of oral bacterial species associated with halitosis. J Am Dent Assoc. 2007;138(8):1113–20.

Hartley MG, El Maaytah MA, McKenzie C, Greenman J. The tongue microbiota of low odour and malodourous individuals. Microbial Ecol Health Dis. 1996;9:215–23.

Hunter CM, Niles HP, Vazquez J, Kloos C, Subramanyam R, Williams MI, Cummins D, Lenton PA, Majerus GJ. Breath odor evaluation by detection of volatile sulfur compounds—correlation with organoleptic odor ratings. Oral Dis. 2005;11(Suppl 1):48–50.

Iwanicka-Grzegorek K, Lipkowska E, Kepa J, Michalik J, Wierzbicka M. Comparison of ninhydrin method of detecting amine compounds with other methods of halitosis detection. Oral Dis. 2005;11(Suppl 1):37–9.

Kleinberg I, Codipilly DM. Cysteine challenge testing: a powerful tool for examining oral malodour processes and treatments in vivo. Int Dent J. 2002;52(Suppl 3):221–8.

Kostelc JG, Zelson PR, Preti G, Tonzetich J. Quantitative differences in volatiles from healthy mouths and mouths with periodontitis. Clin Chem. 1981;27(6):842–5.

Kozlovsky A, Gordon D, Gelernter I, Loesche WJ, Rosenberg M. Correlation between the BANA test and oral malodor parameters. J Dent Res. 1994;73(5):1036–42.

Laleman I, De Geest S, Dekeyser C, Teughels W, Quirynen M. A new method of choice for organoleptic scoring: the negative-pressure technique. J Clin Periodontol. 2018;45(11):1319–25.

Loesche WJ, Bretz WA, Kerschensteiner D, Stoll J, Socransky SS, Hujoel P, Lopatin DE. Development of a diagnostic test for anaerobic periodontal infections based on plaque hydrolysis of benzoyl-DL-arginine-naphthylamide. J Clin Microbiol. 1990;28(7):1551–9.

Mackie RI, Stroot PG, Varel VH. Biochemical identification and biological origin of key odor components in livestock waste. J Anim Sci. 1998;76(5):1331–42.

Masuo Y, Suzuki N, Yoneda M, Naito T, Hirofuji T. Salivary β-galactosidase activity affects physiological oral malodour. Arch Oral Biol. 2012;57(1):87–93.

Morita M, Wang HL. Relationship of sulcular sulfide level to severity of periodontal disease and BANA test. J Periodontol. 2001;72(1):74–8.

Morita M, Musinski DL, Wang HL. Assessment of newly developed tongue sulfide probe for detecting oral malodor. J Clin Periodontol. 2001;28(5):494–6.

Murata T, Yamaga T, Iida T, Miyazaki H, Yaegaki K. Classification and examination of halitosis. Int Dent J. 2002;52(Suppl 3):181–6.

Murata T, Rahardjo A, Fujiyama Y, Yamaga T, Hanada M, Yaegaki K, Miyazaki H. Development of a compact and simple gas chromatography for oral malodor measurement. J Periodontol. 2006;77(7):1142–7.

Nachnani S, Majerus G, Lenton P, Hodges J, Magallanes E. Effects of training on odor judges scoring intensity. Oral Dis. 2005;11(Suppl 1):40–4.

Nonaka A, Tanaka M, Anguri H, Nagata H, Kita J, Shizukuishi S. Clinical assessment of oral malodor intensity expressed as absolute value using an electronic nose. Oral Dis. 2005;11(Suppl 1):35–6.

Oho T, Yoshida Y, Shimazaki Y, Yamashita Y, Koga T. Characteristics of patients complaining of halitosis and the usefulness of gas chromatography for diagnosing halitosis. Oral Surg Oral Med Oral Pathol Oral Radiol Endod. 2001;91(5):531–4.

Petrini M, Trentini P, Ferrante M, D'Alessandro L, Spoto G. Spectrophotometric assessment of salivary β-galactosidases in halitosis. J Breath Res. 2012;6(2):021001.

Petrini M, Costacurta M, Ferrante M, Trentini P, Docimo R, Spoto G. Association between the organoleptic scores, oral condition and salivary β-galactosidases in children affected by halitosis. Int J Dent Hyg. 2014;12(3):213–8.

Pham TA, Ueno M, Shinada K, Kawaguchi Y. Factors affecting oral malodor in periodontitis and gingivitis patients. J Investig Clin Dent. 2012;3(4):284–90.

Quirynen M, Zhao H, Avontroodt P, Soers C, Pauwels M, Coucke W, van Steenberghe D. A salivary incubation test for evaluation of oral malodor: a pilot study. J Periodontol. 2003;74(7):937–44.

Rosenberg M, McCulloch CA. Measurement of oral malodor: current methods and future prospects. J Periodontol. 1992;63(9):776–82.

Rosenberg M, Kulkarni GV, Bosy A, McCulloch CA. Reproducibility and sensitivity of oral malodor measurements with a portable sulphide monitor. J Dent Res. 1991a;70(11):1436–40.

Rosenberg M, Septon I, Eli I, Bar-Ness R, Gelernter I, Brenner S, Gabbay J. Halitosis measurement by an industrial sulphide monitor. J Periodontol. 1991b;62(8):487–9.

Rosenberg M, Knaan T, Cohen D. Association among bad breath, body mass index, and alcohol intake. J Dent Res. 2007;86(10):997–1000.

Schmidt NF, Missan SR, Tarbet WJ. The correlation between organoleptic mouth-odor ratings and levels of volatile sulfur compounds. Oral Surg Oral Med Oral Pathol. 1978;45(4):560–7.

Shimura M, Yasuno Y, Iwakura M, Shimada Y, Sakai S, Suzuki K, Sakamoto S. A new monitor with a zinc-oxide thin film semiconductor sensor for the measurement of volatile sulfur compounds in mouth air. J Periodontol. 1996;67(4):396–402.

Shimura M, Watanabe S, Iwakura M, Oshikiri Y, Kusumoto M, Ikawa K, Sakamoto S. Correlation between measurements using a new halitosis monitor and organoleptic assessment. J Periodontol. 1997;68(12):1182–5.

Solis Gaffar MC, Fischer TJ, Gaffar A. Instrumental evaluation of odor produced by specific oral microorganisms. J Soc Csmet Chem. 1979;30:241–7.

Sopapornamorn P, Ueno M, Vachirarojpisan T, Shinada K, Kawaguchi Y. Association between oral malodor and measurements obtained using a new sulfide monitor. J Dent. 2006;34(10):770–4.

Stamou E, Kozlovsky A, Rosenberg M. Association between Oral malodour and periodontal disease-related parameters in a population of 71 Israelis. Oral Dis. 2005;11(Suppl 1):72–4.

Sterer N, Rosenberg M. Streptococcus salivarius promotes mucin putrefaction and malodor production by Porphyromonas gingivalis. J Dent Res. 2006;85(10):910–4.

Sterer N, Greenstein RB, Rosenberg M. Beta-galactosidase activity in saliva is associated with oral malodor. J Dent Res. 2002;81(3):182–5.

Sterer N, Hendler A, Perez Davidi M, Rosenberg M. A novel microscopic assay for oral malodor related microorganisms. J Breath Res. 2008;2(026003):5pp.

Tamaki N, Kasuyama K, Esaki M, Toshikawa T, Honda S, Ekuni D, Tomofuji T, Morita M. A new portable monitor for measuring odorous compounds in oral, exhaled and nasal air. BMC Oral Health. 2011;11:15.

Tanaka M, Anguri H, Nonaka A, Kataoka K, Nagata H, Kita J, Shizukuishi S. Clinical assessment of oral malodor by the electronic nose system. J Dent Res. 2004a;83(4):317–21.

Tanaka M, Yamamoto Y, Kuboniwa M, Nonaka A, Nishida N, Maeda K, Kataoka K, Nagata H, Shizukuishi S. Contribution of periodontal pathogens on tongue dorsa analyzed with real-time PCR to oral malodor. Microbes Infect. 2004b;6(12):1078–83.

Tonzetich J. Direct gas chromatographic analysis of sulphur compounds in mouth air in man. Arch Oral Biol. 1971;16(6):587–97.

Tonzetich J, Carpenter PA. Production of volatile sulphur compounds from cysteine, cystine and methionine by human dental plague. Arch Oral Biol. 1971;16(6):599–607.

Ueno M, Takeuchi S, Samnieng P, Morishima S, Shinada K, Kawaguchi Y. Turbidity of mouth-rinsed water as a screening index for oral malodor. Oral Surg Oral Med Oral Pathol Oral Radiol. 2013;116(2):203–9.

Vandekerckhove B, Van den Velde S, De Smit M, Dadamio J, Teughels W, Van Tornout M, Quirynen M. Clinical reliability of non-organoleptic oral malodour measurements. J Clin Periodontol. 2009;36(11):964–9.

Wåler SM. On the transformation of sulfur containing amino acids and peptides to volatile sulfur compounds (vsc) in the human mouth. Eur J Oral Sci. 1997;105:534–7.

Willis CL, Gibson GR, Holt J, Allison C. Negative correlation between oral malodour and numbers and activities of sulphate-reducing bacteria in the human mouth. Arch Oral Biol. 1999;44(8):665–70.

Yaegaki K, Sanada K. Volatile sulfur compounds in mouth air from clinically healthy subjects and patients with periodontal disease. J Periodontal Res. 1992;27(4 Pt 1):233–8.

Yoneda M, Masuo Y, Suzuki N, Iwamoto T, Hirofuji T. Relationship between the β-galactosidase activity in saliva and parameters associated with oral malodor. J Breath Res. 2010;4(1):017108 (6pp).

Breath Odor Diagnosis

9

Contents

Unlike other complaints such as pain, discomfort, or impaired esthetics, breath odors are not sensed by the patients themselves but rather by their close environment (e.g., friends, family members, coworkers). As a result, patients are unable to give a reliable report on their condition (e.g., onset, frequency, duration, intensity). Therefore, it is important to make sure that the patient brings a family member or a close friend ("confidant") to the appointment (Rosenberg 1996).

Additionally, modern society is constantly exposed to commercial advertisements stressing the importance of fresh breath, fueling excessive worry surrounding this issue, also known as halitophobia (for more details, see Chap. 12). One result of this phenomenon is that about 20% of the patients complaining of breath odors present in the clinic without any appreciable odor that can be objectively detected (Quirynen et al. 2009; Seemann et al. 2006).

The first diagnostic challenge in the clinic is to confirm whether or not the patient is suffering from an objective malodor problem, referred to by some researchers as genuine halitosis (Yaegaki and Coil 2000).

9.1 Pre-appointment Instructions

In order to enable the clinician to properly diagnose breath odor problems patients should avoid any malodor-mitigating activities such as eating, drinking, or gum chewing for 2–3 h prior to their appointment (Rosenberg 1996). Avoiding eating or drinking for longer periods of time (e.g., 6–12 h) has been suggested in the literature (Murata et al. 2002; Richter 1996). However, such a restriction may be problematic in the case of small children or diabetic patients, does not imitate normal everyday life and may lead to overdiagnosis and overtreatment.

Since malodor production is due to bacterial activity, malodor diagnosis should not be performed during or immediately following antibiotic treatment. If the patient is receiving antibiotics, diagnosis should be postponed till 3–4 weeks posttreatment. Performing malodor diagnosis during or immediately following antibiotic treatment may result in misdiagnosing a patient actually suffering from the problem.

On the day of examination patients should maintain their regular everyday oral hygiene activity. However, these activities should not include mouthrinse use and should not be performed within 2–3 h prior to the appointment to avoid malodor reduction.

To minimize contribution of extraneous odor sources, the consumption of onion, garlic, alcoholic beverages, coffee as well as smoking should be avoided for 12 h prior to the appointment. Scented lipstick, cologne, or perfumes should not be worn on the day of examination, as they might affect odor judge assessment.

9.2 Patient Interview

Due to the sensitive nature of the subject patient interviewing should be done discretely in a private setting (Lenton et al. 2001). A fruitful discussion on the subject can only be carried out in a calm relaxed atmosphere where trust can be established.

In some cases, the patient's chief complaint is self-perceived malodor, which often relies on either oral discomfort (e.g., bad taste, dryness) or the patient's interpretation of others' behavior (e.g., head averting, nose covering, and stepping back; see also Chaps. 10 and 12). It is important to stress that these sensations are often unassociated with malodor and that reliable information regarding breath odor problems (e.g., onset, frequency, duration, intensity) is best provided by a "confidant," i.e., family member or a close friend of the patient (Rosenberg 1996) who is aware of the actual problem.

A complete medical history should be taken to rule out any possible systemic or ENT conditions or medications that may contribute or cause malodor. Dental history should also be taken with an emphasis on oral hygiene practice including frequency of tooth brushing, flossing, tongue cleaning, and mouthrinsing. Special attention should be given to habits of smoking, alcohol, and coffee consumption and eating habits (e.g., avoiding breakfast). Factors such as mouth breathing (e.g., snoring) and insufficient fluid intake should also be addressed, as they can promote oral dryness. Allergic reactions, specifically in the form of allergic rhinitis (sneezing and "running nose"), may cause increased postnasal drip.

9.3 Examination

9.3.1 Organoleptic Measurements

In order to assess the severity of the problem, the clinician should instruct the patient to refrain from talking for 5 min. Then, the patient is asked to exhale through the mouth or talk (e.g., "count to 20") and the clinician rates the malodor intensity on his breath using a 0–5 grading scale (Rosenberg et al. 1991) from a set distance of 10 cm. It is very important that the clinician perform a repeated "sniffing" action to allow the chemical component of the malodor to be more easily detected (Greenman et al. 2014). Next, the patient is instructed to exhale through the nose and malodor is again evaluated in the same manner.

If the malodor comes primarily from the mouth, an oral or pharyngeal etiology may be suspected and a thorough examination of the oral cavity is warranted. If however, the malodor comes primarily from the nose a nasal etiology is more likely and the patient should be referred to an ENT specialist. In rare cases in which the malodor is similar in quality and intensity from both the mouth and the nose a systemic or external etiology may be the main cause.

In some cases, no malodor is apparent and the problem cannot be confirmed. In these cases, when a close friend or family member maintains that there is an odor problem the examination should be repeated on a different occasion, preferably in the late afternoon or late morning hours (Miyazaki et al. 1995). Otherwise, if malodor cannot be detected then halitophobia may be the most likely cause for the patient's complaint.

9.3.2 Oral VSC Quantification

The instrumental quantification of volatile sulfide compounds within the oral cavity is an important adjunct tool in oral malodor research and diagnosis. It enables the clinician to record and present to the patient a measurable objective parameter associated with the malodor. This helps either to confirm or rule out the existence of a malodor problem as defined organoleptically by the odor judge, as well as following treatment outcome.

The most commonly used instrument for quantitative measurements has been the portable sulfide monitor (i.e., Halimeter™). Its simple use, low maintenance, quick response, and portability make it an applicable instrument for both research and the clinic. Its major disadvantages are its sensitivity to high levels of other compounds (e.g., alcohol) and its inability to distinguish between various volatile sulfide compounds.

Gas chromatography (GC) has been used since the early 1970s as the method of choice for measuring individual sulfide gases present in mouth air samples. However, this technique requires high technical skills and maintenance. Recently, a more simple to use instrument was devised based on GC technology (i.e., OralChroma™; Murata et al. 2006). However, whereas some clinicians attribute diagnostic value to the differentiation between the various volatile sulfides, this claim remains under dispute. Therefore, most researchers and clinicians agree that although GC measurements are more suitable to research, total VSC measurement using a simple sulfide monitor appears to be more appropriate for the clinical setting (Laleman et al. 2014).

9.3.3 Examination of the Oral Cavity

In cases where an oral etiology is suspected a thorough examination of the oral cavity is warranted. This should include the tongue, gingival, and periodontal tissues as well as clinical and radiographical examination of the teeth.

When examining the tongue, special attention should be given to the presence and extent of tongue coating. The extent of the tongue coating can be either scored and recorded using a simple tongue coating index based on coating area and/or thickness (for more details, see Chap. 2), or by digital images analysis (Kim et al. 2009). Following scoring, tongue coating can be sampled using swab, gauze pad, brush, or plastic spoon sampling of the posterior dorsal tongue ("spoon test"; Rosenberg 1996). It is important to make sure that the sample is obtained from the very back of the tongue. This can be done by holding the tip of the extended tongue using a gauze pad with one hand and sampling with the other. Then the malodor emanating from this sample can be scored organoleptically (e.g., 0–5 scale) and compared to the character of the overall odor (both by the clinician and the confidant).

Patients should be checked for the presence of periodontal pockets of 5 mm or more and gingival index as well as plaque index should be recorded. Special attention should be given to sites with signs of active inflammation (i.e., bleeding on probing). An interdental plaque sample from these sites can be obtained using regular unscented dental floss, special floss (e.g., Superfloss™), or an interdental brush. These samples can also be scored organoleptically (e.g., 0–5 scale) and compared to the overall quality of the oral odor.

Clinical and radiographical examination of the teeth should be conducted in order to identify any possible contributing factors including faulty dental restorations (e.g., overhanging margins, food impaction sites, caries lesions), and leaky crowns (e.g., decemented crowns). Removable dentures should be evaluated separately outside of the oral cavity. This could be done by placing them for a few minutes in a closed plastic bag and evaluating the malodor produced (Rosenberg 1996).

9.3.4 Biochemical and Microbial Assays

The growing body of knowledge accumulated over the last decades regarding the microbial and biochemical processes involved in malodor production has led to the development of several auxiliary diagnostic assays that can be implemented in the clinic (i.e., "chair side").

These assays play a role in providing additional quantitatively measurable malodor-related parameters for the clinician as well as providing an important tool for patient education.

Biochemical assays (e.g., BANA test, β-galactosidase assay) are enzymatic-based assays typically producing a color response as a result of an enzymatic activity related to the malodor production process (e.g., proteolysis, deglycosylation). These color tests are relatively rapid and enable the visualization and quantification of an otherwise abstract notion such as malodor production. Furthermore, these assays offer additional corroboration for the diagnosis of the suspected malodor origin and etiology.

Microbial assays are less commonly used because they usually require additional equipment and prolonged incubation. However, some clinicians do utilize live microscopy (e.g., wet mount, phase microscopy) to demonstrate to the patient the bacterial nature and abundance of plaque samples taken from various locations in the mouth (e.g., teeth, tongue).

References

Greenman J, Lenton P, Seemann R, Nachnani S. Organoleptic assessment of halitosis for dental professionals—general recommendations. J Breath Res. 2014;8(1):017102.

Kim J, Jung Y, Park K, Park JW. A digital tongue imaging system for tongue coating evaluation in patients with oral malodour. Oral Dis. 2009;15(8):565–9.

Laleman I, Dadamio J, De Geest S, Dekeyser C, Quirynen M. Instrumental assessment of halitosis for the general dental practitioner. J Breath Res. 2014;8(1):017103.

Lenton P, Majerus G, Bakdash B. Counseling and treating bad breath patients: a step-by-step approach. J Contemp Dent Pract. 2001;2(2):46–61.

Miyazaki H, Sakao S, Katoh Y, Takehara T. Correlation between volatile sulphur compounds and certain oral health measurements in the general population. J Periodontol. 1995;66(8):679–84.

Murata T, Yamaga T, Iida T, Miyazaki H, Yaegaki K. Classification and examination of halitosis. Int Dent J. 2002;52(Suppl 3):181–6.

Murata T, Rahardjo A, Fujiyama Y, Yamaga T, Hanada M, Yaegaki K, Miyazaki H. Development of a compact and simple gas chromatography for oral malodor measurement. J Periodontol. 2006;77(7):1142–7.

Quirynen M, Dadamio J, Van den Velde S, De Smit M, Dekeyser C, Van Tornout M, Vandekerckhove B. Characteristics of 2000 patients who visited a halitosis clinic. J Clin Periodontol. 2009;36(11):970–5.

Richter JL. Diagnosis and treatment of halitosis. Compend Contin Educ Dent. 1996;17(4):370–2, 374–6 passim; quiz 388.

Rosenberg M. Clinical assessment of bad breath: current concepts. J Am Dent Assoc. 1996;127(4):475–82.

Rosenberg M, Kulkarni GV, Bosy A, McCulloch CA. Reproducibility and sensitivity of oral malodor measurements with a portable sulphide monitor. J Dent Res. 1991;70(11):1436–40.

Seemann R, Bizhang M, Djamchidi C, Kage A, Nachnani S. The proportion of pseudo-halitosis patients in a multidisciplinary breath malodour consultation. Int Dent J. 2006;56(2):77–81.

Yaegaki K, Coil JM. Examination, classification, and treatment of halitosis; clinical perspectives. J Can Dent Assoc. 2000;66(5):257–61.

Self-Assessment of Breath Odors

10

Content

The inability of a person to sense his own breath results in a situation called the "bad breath paradox" (Scott Harper, personal communication). According to this paradox many people suffering from breath odors are unaware of their condition, whereas many others that do not have any breath odor worry excessively that they do. For example, in a study of 88 subjects attending a routine health checkup, 19 thought that they had bad breath, but this was not confirmed by the odor judge. Conversely, nine had confirmed breath odor but were not aware of it (Rosenberg et al. 2007). In another study conducted in Japan (Iwakura et al. 1994), 80% of the patients who visited the clinic claimed to be self-aware of their condition, while only 24% had actual malodor.

Some researchers attributed the inability to sense one's own breath to olfactory accommodation or adaptation (Spouge 1964), i.e. continuous exposure to an odor stimuli resulting in specific desensitization of the olfactory system to that odorant. However, research indicates that this may not be the case, since subjects were able to sense the malodor of their saliva (Greenstein et al. 1997; Rosenberg et al. 1995) even though this malodor ostensibly comprises many of the same odorants. Therefore, it seems that the expla-nation for this phenomenon is much simpler. Since bad breath usually emanates from the mouth during exhalation and speech, the malodor components are largely diluted into the air by the time the subjects re-inhales them the through the nose. This drop in concentration of volatiles may result in levels that are below detection. This may be why people cannot detect their own breath odors while the people facing them can.

Most researchers found no correlations between self-reported breath odor ratings and breath odor objective clinical measurements as carried out by the trained odor judge (Bornstein et al. 2009; Rosenberg et al. 1995) and therefore concluded that self-reported breath odor is an unreliable parameter. One study on the other hand did conclude that "self-estimation of bad breath correlated well with the presence of oral malodor" (Romano et al. 2010). However, a critical review of the results of this study shows no correlation between the self-assessment and the odor judge ratings or other clinical parameters. Despite these facts many studies still erro-neously rely on self-reported breath odors, usually by means of a questionnaire as an objective parameter in breath odor investigations (e.g., see Chap. 6).

It seems that the physical inability to detect one's breath odor is not the only limitation in self-assessment of breath odors. Research showed that even when given a sample of their odor (e.g., tongue coating sample) subjects lacked the ability to objectively rate and score the odor. It seems that there are psychological factors that color our objectivity about our own body traits, including smells. For example, in 1995, a study was reported on self-assessment of bad breath involving 52 subjects, 43 of whom were concerned that they did have bad breath (Rosenberg et al. 1995). They were asked to fill out a questionnaire, asking them to score their own oral malodor as follows:

(a) Preconception score—prior to measurement, subjects were asked to score the level of bad breath which they thought they had at that time;

(b) Mouth odor—subjects were asked to cup their hands over their mouth and nose, exhale through the mouth and breath in through the nose, and subsequently score the odor.

(c) Tongue odor—subjects were asked to lick their wrist and smell and score that odor.

(d) Saliva odor—subjects were asked to smell and score their own saliva, placed in a plastic dish.

(e) Post-measurement score—subjects were asked to again rate their own odor, following all three self-tests.

All these subjects and samples were also scored by an experienced odor judge.

The results of this study showed that with the exception of saliva, subjects' self-assessments were completely unrelated to odor judge scores, volatile sulfides, cadaverine, or oral status. Instead, they remained closely associated with their preconception scores. Even after the three attempts at smelling their own malodor, the post-measurement scores remained unassociated with any of the objective parameters, yet highly associated with the subjective preconception score ($R = 0.72$, $P < 0.001$).

One year following the initial experiment, 32 of the concerned subjects were invited back to the laboratory for a follow-up assessment (Rosenberg

et al. 1999). Although the mouth odor and saliva odor of the subjects had significantly improved according to the odor judge, $p = 0.006$ and $p = 0.009$, respectively (they had been given instructions during the initial study 1 year prior and 85% had sought dental care), the subjects' self-assessments of mouth odor and saliva odor showed no significant improvement ($p = 0.22$ and $p = 0.50$, respectively). Instead, they seemed to sense a slight but significant improvement in tongue odor ($p = 0.017$), which was not supported by the objective odor judge ($p = 0.98$). Their self-assessment of tongue odor was closely associated again with their preconception of how bad they thought the odor would be ($r = 0.65$, $p < 0.001$), and how they scored it at the initial consultation ($r = 0.71$, $p < 0.001$). None of the self-scores were significantly related to any of the odor judge scores. Another study conducted on 565 dental patients (Pham et al. 2012) concluded that self-perception was an invalid method for evaluating one's breath yielding low sensitivity and specificity (47 and 59%, respectively). Furthermore, self-reported breath odors were associated with smoking and alcohol consumption but not with any of the objective clinical parameters such as odor judge scores, gingivitis, and tongue coating.

It appears that subjects who are concerned about having breath odors tend to give their breath samples higher scores as compared to the objective scores given the odor judge (Eli et al. 2001). Subjects recruited for reasons other than breath concerns may exhibit higher levels of overall agreement with objective parameters. For example, among the 88 subjects attending a routine medical checkup, self-reporting of halitosis as compared with odor judge scoring (at a cutoff of greater than or equal to 2) yielded an accuracy of 67%. Other researchers also reported that in the majority of cases, the patient's own assessment was higher than the organoleptic assessment and suggested a psychological basis for this phenomenon (Dudzik et al. 2015).

In another study (Nalcaci and Baran 2008), 254 "healthy elderly" Turkish subjects (mean age 62) were asked regarding their oral health status. Among them 28% reported that they suffered from bad breath. Most of these subjects also reported oral dryness (74%). Although each subject underwent a comprehensive dental examination, including tongue coating level, the researchers did not actually smell the odor of the subjects, nor did they perform any adjunct testing for VSC levels. Nevertheless, a significant and relatively high correlation between self-reported bad breath and tongue coating levels ($p = 0.59$, $p = 0.0001$) was recorded, followed by self-reported oral dryness ($p = 0.41$, $p = 0.0001$). Other researchers also reported the association between the discomfort brought about by oral dryness and higher levels of self-reported halitosis in Parkinson's patients, when in fact these xerostomic patients showed much lower levels of oral malodor as compared with the control group (Barbe et al. 2017).

Self-assessment of breath odors appears to be associated with various factors such as lack of good oral hygiene, smoking, presence of tongue coating, subjective and objective oral dryness, wearing dentures, gum disease, alcohol consumption age (over 30), and gender (females) (Al-Ansari et al. 2006; Nalcaci and Baran 2008; Settineri et al. 2010). Females seem to give themselves higher malodor scores than men. For instance, one study reported that women scored significantly higher than men in rating their own malodor although men were assigned higher scores by the odor judge. In that study, 25 out of 88 women gave themselves the highest score of "5" (on a 0–5 scale) as compared to "3.5" given by the odor judge. Nevertheless, self-estimates of both genders were still significantly higher than odor judge scores (Rosenberg and Leib 1997).

References

Al-Ansari JM, Boodai H, Al-Sumait N, Al-Khabbaz AK, Al-Shammari KF, Salako N. Factors associated with self-reported halitosis in Kuwaiti patients. J Dent. 2006;34(7):444–9.

Barbe AG, Deutscher DHC, Derman SHM, Hellmich M, Noack MJ. Subjective and objective halitosis among patients with Parkinson's disease. Gerodontology. 2017;34(4):460–8.

Bornstein MM, Stocker BL, Seemann R, Burgin WB, Lussi A. Prevalence of halitosis in young male adults: a study in swiss army recruits comparing self-reported and clinical data. J Periodontol. 2009;80(1):24–31.

Dudzik A, Chomyszyn-Gajewska M, Łazarz-Bartyzel K. An evaluation of halitosis using oral chroma™ data manager, organoleptic scores and patients' subjective opinions. J Int Oral Health. 2015;7(3):6–11.

Eli I, Baht R, Koriat H, Rosenberg M. Self-perception of breath odor. J Am Dent Assoc. 2001;132(5):621–6.

Greenstein RB, Goldberg S, Marku-Cohen S, Sterer N, Rosenberg M. Reduction of oral malodor by oxidizing lozenges. J Periodontol. 1997;68(12):1176–81.

Iwakura M, Yasuno Y, Shimura M, Sakamoto S. Clinical characteristics of halitosis: differences in two patient groups with primary and secondary complaints of halitosis. J Dent Res. 1994;73(9):1568–74.

Nalcaci R, Baran I. Factors associated with self-reported halitosis (SRH) and perceived taste disturbance (PTD) in elderly. Arch Gerontol Geriatr. 2008;46(3):307–16.

Pham TA, Ueno M, Shinada K, Kawaguchi Y. Comparison between self-perceived and clinical oral malodor. Oral Surg Oral Med Oral Pathol Oral Radiol. 2012;113(1):70–80.

Romano F, Pigella E, Guzzi N, Aimetti M. Patients' self-assessment of oral malodour and its relationship with organoleptic scores and oral conditions. Int J Dent Hyg. 2010;8(1):41–6.

Rosenberg M, Leib E. Experiences of an Israeli malodor clinic. In: Rosenberg M, editor. Bad breath research perspectives. Tel Aviv: Ramot Publishing—Tel Aviv University; 1997. p. 137–48.

Rosenberg M, Kozlovsky A, Gelernter I, Cherniak O, Gabbay J, Baht R, Eli I. Self-estimation of oral malodor. J Dent Res. 1995;74(9):1577–82.

Rosenberg M, Kozlovsky A, Wind Y, Mindel E. Self-assessment of oral malodor 1 year following initial consultation. Quintessence Int. 1999;30(5):324–7.

Rosenberg M, Knaan T, Cohen D. Association among bad breath, body mass index, and alcohol intake. J Dent Res. 2007;86(10):997–1000.

Settineri S, Mento C, Gugliotta SC, Saitta A, Terranova A, Trimarchi G, Mallamace D. Self-reported halitosis and emotional state: impact on oral conditions and treatments. Health Qual Life Outcomes. 2010;8:34.

Spouge JD. Halitosis: a review of its causes and treatment. Dent Pract. 1964;14:307–17.

Breath Odors, Prevalence, Gender, and Age

Contents

11.1 Prevalence

Breath odors are a common condition. Various studies conducted around the world in different populations, using odor judge and instrumental measuring techniques and with varying threshold criteria have found prevalence of bad breath to range from as low as 2% of the population to over 60% (Table 11.1). It is clear that the lack of standardization in threshold criteria and measuring techniques is a major cause for this large variation. One study conducted in Sweden (Soder et al. 2000) used strong, noticeably unpleasant odor (i.e., "Foetor ex ore") as the criterion for breath odors. In this study the researchers reported a prevalence of 2.4% in a population of 1681 subjects. Using such a high threshold that is equivalent to an odor judge score of "4" (i.e. "strong malodor") on a 0–5 scale yielded a similarly low prevalence (2.14%) in a study done in Swaziland (Bornstein et al. 2009). However, in the same study, when an odor judge score of "2" and above was considered the threshold for malodor (i.e., "mild, clearly noticeable malodor") prevalence reached 31.5%.

Indeed, most studies use "slight but noticeable" (i.e., odor judge scores of "2" on a 0–5 scale) as the threshold value for breath odors (Bornstein et al. 2009; Iwanicka-Grzegorek et al. 2005; Liu et al. 2006; Rosenberg et al. 2007). When this criterion is applied, prevalence is consistently found to be in the range 27.5–31.5%.

A few studies based their breath odor assessment solely on oral VSC levels (Miyazaki et al. 1995, 1997) as measured using a sulfide monitor (i.e., Halimeter), whereas others used VSC measurements adjunct to organoleptic scorings (Bornstein et al. 2009; Iwanicka-Grzegorek et al. 2005; Liu et al. 2006). These studies regarded different VSC concentration values as cutoff points for breath odor conformation (e.g., 75, 110, 125 ppb, respectively). It is important to stress that although VSC readings using Halimeter are in high correlation with organoleptic scores and their value is an important parameter for clinical follow-up, the absolute value of a given reading can vary between different instruments depending on the sensor's sensitivity and calibration. Therefore, setting a universal cutoff value would be impractical.

© Springer Nature Switzerland AG 2020

N. Sterer, M. Rosenberg, *Breath Odors*, https://doi.org/10.1007/978-3-030-44731-1_11

Table 11.1 Prevalence of breath odors

References	Subjects population	Malodor parameter	Criteria/cutoff	Prevalence (%)
Sulser et al. (1939)	$n = 200$ Age n.d.	Osmoscope (indirect method)	Malodor score of PO_2 and above ("objectionable")	56
Morris and Read (1949)	No. n.d. Age 18–60 years	Osmoscope (direct method; 2 operators)	Malodor score of PO_3 and above (1–6) ("halitosis")	65
Miyazaki et al. (1995)	$n = 2672$ Age 18–64 years	VSC measured by Halimeter	VSC level ≥ 75 ppb Less than 2 h following meals. More than 2 h following meals	6–14 16–23
Miyazaki et al. (1997)	$n = 2601$ Age 18–64 years	VSC measured by Halimeter	VSC level ≥ 75 ppb Less than 2.5 h following meals. More than 2.5 h following meals	8–15 18–25
Loesche et al. (1996)	$n = 270$ Age ≥ 60 years	Questionnaire	"Been told you have" "Think you have"	24 31
Soder et al. (2000)	$n = 1681$ Mean age 36 years	Organoleptic	Strong, noticeably unpleasant odor ("Foetor ex ore")	2.4
Iwanicka-Grzegorek et al. (2005)	$n = 295$ Age 18–74 years	Organoleptic Halimeter	Malodor score ≥ 2 (0–5) VSC levels ≥ 125 ppb	29.7 24.5
Liu et al. (2006)	$n = 2000$ Age 15–64 years	Organoleptic Halimeter	Malodor score ≥ 2 (0–5) VSC levels ≥ 75 ppb ≥ 110 ppb	27.5 35.4 20.3
Nadanovsky et al. (2007)	$n = 344$ Age 1–87 years	Informants questionnaire	"Yes" to: "Family member with bad breath?"	15
Rosenberg et al. (2007)	$n = 88$ (46 M) Age 20–55 years	Organoleptic	Malodor score ≥ 2 (0–5)	29.8
Bornstein et al. (2009)	$n = 419$ Age 18–94 years	Organoleptic Halimeter	Malodor score ≥ 2 (0–5) ≥ 3 (0–5) ≥ 4 (0–5) VSC levels ≥ 75 ppb ≥ 110 ppb	31.5 11.4 2.14 27.9
Chen et al. (2016)	$n = 720$ (347 M) Age 22–70 years	Halimeter	VSC levels ≥ 110 ppb	33.2

11.2   Gender

Gender is usually not taken into account in breath odor investigations since most studies report no difference between male and female subjects in the prevalence or levels of malodor (Miyazaki et al. 1995; Sulser et al. 1939). However, as shown in Table 11.2, some studies did report a variation between males and females. One study conducted in the general population of China (Liu et al. 2006) showed elevated VSC levels in females in the age group of 35–44 years as compared to males. Although this study did not find similar results in the other age groups it has been reported in the literature that women showed a two- to fourfold increase in VSC levels in mouth air during and shortly prior to menstruation (Calil et al. 2008; Tonzetich et al. 1978) especially in

women with signs of periodontal disease (Kawamoto et al. 2010). This increase in VSC levels coincided with hormonal levels and salivary flow reduction.

On the other hand, studies conducted in Brazil and Italy reported higher prevalence of breath odors in males as compared to females (Nadanovsky et al. 2007; Aimetti et al. 2015), although one of these studies relied on questionnaire reports by a family member rather than actual measurements.

11.3   Age

Although some researchers reported an increase in breath odors with age (Sulser et al. 1939; Aimetti et al. 2015), most studies conducted on

Table 11.2 Gender, age, and breath odors

References	Subjects	Gender	Age
Sulser et al. (1939)	n = 200 (64% males) Age groups: ≤20 (n = 20) 21–50 (n = 144) ≥51 (n = 36)	Equal prevalence in males and females (on average)	Malodor increased with age
Miyazaki et al. (1995)	n = 2672 (64% males) Age groups: 15–24 (n = 317) 25–34 (n = 595) 35–44 (n = 916) 45–54 (n = 615) 55–64 (n = 229)	No difference in VSC levels between males and females	No difference in VSC levels between age groups
Liu et al. (2006)	n = 2000 (50% males) Age groups: 15–24 (n = 400) 25–34 (n = 400) 35–44 (n = 400) 45–54 (n = 400) 55–64 (n = 400)	Significantly higher VSC level in females in age group 35–44 years correlations between gender and VSC levels (logistic regression analysis)	No difference in VSC levels between age groups
Nadanovsky et al. (2007)	n = 344 (49% males) Age 1–87 years (mean 39 ± 18)	Higher prevalence in males (21%) then females (9%)	Higher prevalence in people over 20 years old (17%) then under 20 years old (7%) for both sexes
Patil et al. (2014)	n = 900 school children (7–15 years)	No association between malodor and gender	Association between malodor levels and age. Average malodor prevalence 41%
Villa et al. (2014)	n = 101 children and adolescents (6–16 years) Age groups: 6–12 (n = 44) 13–16 (n = 57)	Higher prevalence in females (58%) than males (42%)	Higher prevalence in adolescents age group (VSC > 100 ppb): 32% 68%
Aimetti et al. (2015)	n = 744 (42% males) Age groups: 20–29 (n = 80) 30–39 (n = 116) 40–49 (n = 159) 50–59 (n = 193) 60–75 (n = 196)	Higher prevalence in males (61%) then females (51%)	Higher prevalence ($p < 0.001$) with age: 32% 44% 49% 65% 65%
Zellmer et al. (2016)	n = 124 nursing home residents (23% males) Age 66–99 (mean age 86.9)	No difference in malodor prevalence between genders	High prevalence of malodor in elderly living in nursing homes (54%)
Ueno et al. (2018)	n = 768 school children (6–15 years) (54% males)	No difference in malodor prevalence between genders	Higher malodor prevalence in seventh to ninth grade (49%) than first to third grade (36%)

adult populations did not find age to be a risk factor (Table 11.2). Nevertheless, several recent studies conducted in various places around the world on the prevalence of breath odors in school children, adolescents, and elderly population (Patil et al. 2014; Villa et al. 2014; Zellmer et al. 2016; Ueno et al. 2018) reported relatively high prevalence rates (ranging between 41 and 68%)

as compared with previous reports (Nadanovsky et al. 2007) and the general population.

Whether or not age plays a part in the prevalence and severity of this problem is yet to be determined. However, it is clear that the origins of oral malodor and its character may vary with age. In children and adolescents, oral malodor is mainly associated with tongue coating scores (Amir et al. 1999; Nalcaci and Sonmez 2008; Ueno et al. 2018). Nevertheless, studies have shown a significant increase in malodor-related parameters in adolescents as compared with younger children (Villa et al. 2014; Ueno et al. 2018) a possible explanation for this observation is the frequent use of fixed orthodontic appliances in that age group and its association with malodor production (for more details, see Chap. 2). Whereas, the tongue seems to play a major role in oral malodor throughout life, other factors may add on and vary. For example, after the age of 45 periodontal disease becomes associated with malodor production (Bosy et al. 1994). Taking various medications may affect saliva flow in subjects over the age of 50 (e.g., antihypertensive drugs), and in the elderly population denture-related problems may contribute to malodor production. In a recent study conducted on elderly population residing in nursing homes in Sweden a high prevalence of 54% of breath odors was reported as associated with hyposalivation and dementia (Zellmer et al. 2016).

In summary, future studies looking at different age groups should assess not only odor intensity, but the quality of the odor, as well as its source (e.g., mouth vs. nose, dentures vs. permanent dentition) especially when looking for correlations between odor and age-specific parameters.

References

Aimetti M, Perotto S, Castiglione A, Ercoli E, Romano F. Prevalence estimation of halitosis and its association with oral health-related parameters in an adult population of a city in North Italy. J Clin Periodontol. 2015;42(12):1105–14.

Amir E, Shimonov R, Rosenberg M. Halitosis in children. J Pediatr. 1999;134(3):338–43.

Bornstein MM, Kislig K, Hoti BB, Seemann R, Lussi A. Prevalence of halitosis in the population of the city of Bern, Switzerland: a study comparing self-reported and clinical data. Eur J Oral Sci. 2009;117(3):261–7.

Bosy A, Kulkarni GV, Rosenberg M, McCulloch CA. Relationship of oral malodor to periodontitis: evidence of independence in discrete subpopulations. J Periodontol. 1994;65(1):37–46.

Calil CM, Lima PO, Bernardes CF, Groppo FC, Bado F, Marcondes FK. Influence of gender and menstrual cycle on volatile sulphur compounds production. Arch Oral Biol. 2008;53(12):1107–12.

Chen X, Zhang Y, Lu HX, Feng XP. Factors associated with halitosis in white-collar employees in Shanghai, China. PLoS One. 2016;11(5):e0155592.

Iwanicka-Grzegorek E, Michalik J, Kepa J, Wierzbicka M, Aleksinski M, Pierzynowska E. Subjective patients' opinion and evaluation of halitosis using halimeter and organoleptic scores. Oral Dis. 2005;11(Suppl 1):86–8.

Kawamoto A, Sugano N, Motohashi M, Matsumoto S, Ito K. Relationship between oral malodor and the menstrual cycle. J Periodontal Res. 2010;45(5):681–7.

Liu XN, Shinada K, Chen XC, Zhang BX, Yaegaki K, Kawaguchi Y. Oral malodor-related parameters in the Chinese general population. J Clin Periodontol. 2006;33(1):31–6.

Loesche WJ, Grossman N, Dominguez L, Schork A. Oral malodour in the elderly. In: Van Steenberghe D, Rosenberg M, editors. Bad breath a multidisciplinary approach. Leuven: Leuven University Press; 1996. p. 181–94.

Miyazaki H, Sakao S, Katoh Y, Takehara T. Correlation between volatile sulphur compounds and certain oral health measurements in the general population. J Periodontol. 1995;66(8):679–84.

Miyazaki H, Sakao S, Katoh Y, Takehara T. Oral malodor in the general population of Japan. In: Rosenberg M, editor. Bad breath research perspectives. Tel Aviv: Ramot Publishing—Tel Aviv University; 1997. p. 118–36.

Morris PP, Read RR. Halitosis; variations in mouth and total breath odor intensity resulting from prophylaxis and antisepsis. J Dent Res. 1949;28(3):324–33.

Nadanovsky P, Carvalho LB, Ponce de Leon A. Oral malodour and its association with age and sex in a general population in Brazil. Oral Dis. 2007;13(1):105–9.

Nalcaci R, Sonmez IS. Evaluation of oral malodor in children. Oral Surg Oral Med Oral Pathol Oral Radiol Endod. 2008;106(3):384–8.

Patil PS, Pujar P, Poornima S, Subbareddy VV. Prevalence of oral malodour and its relationship with oral parameters in Indian children aged 7-15 years. Eur Arch Paediatr Dent. 2014;15(4):251–8.

Rosenberg M, Knaan T, Cohen D. Association among bad breath, body mass index, and alcohol intake. J Dent Res. 2007;86(10):997–1000.

Soder B, Johansson B, Soder PO. The relation between foetor ex ore, oral hygiene and periodontal disease. Swed Dent J. 2000;24(3):73–82.

Sulser GF, Brening RH, Fosdick LS. Some conditions that effect the odor concentration of breath. J Dent Res. 1939;18(4):355–9.

Tonzetich J, Preti G, Huggins GR. Changes in concentration of volatile sulphur compounds of mouth air during the menstrual cycle. J Int Med Res. 1978;6(3):245–54.

Ueno M, Ohnuki M, Zaitsu T, Takehara S, Furukawa S, Kawaguchi Y. Prevalence and risk factors of halitosis in Japanese school children. Pediatr Int. 2018;60(6):588–92.

Villa A, Zollanvari A, Alterovitz G, Cagetti MG, Strohmenger L, Abati S. Prevalence of halitosis in children considering oral hygiene, gender and age. Int J Dent Hyg. 2014;12(3):208–12.

Zellmer M, Gahnberg L, Ramberg P. Prevalence of halitosis in elderly living in nursing homes. Int J Dent Hyg. 2016;14(4):295–300.

Psychological Aspects of Breath Odors

12

Contents

12.1   Halitophobia

In some 15–30% of patients complaining of a serious breath odor problem, little or no malodor can be detected by the examiner either organolepticaly by smelling the patient's breath or using laboratory techniques (Quirynen et al. 2009; Seemann et al. 2006). These patients vary in their level of conviction regarding their perceived odor problem. Some just wish to confirm or rule out a breath odor problem, whereas others firmly believe that the problem exists. In extreme cases patients may appear psychotic and/or contemplate suicide (Yaegaki and Coil 1999). In 1995, we coined the term "halitophobic" to describe patients with a complaint of halitosis that cannot be verified. Some researchers have dichotomously subclassified these patients into "Pseudo halitosis" and "Halitophobia" based on their treatment response and need of psychiatric consultation (Yaegaki and Coil 2000). Alternatively, other researchers regard "Halitophobia" as a "mild to severe" spectrum of conditions that include any level of exaggerated concern over having a breath odor problem (Rosenberg and Leib 1997).

Convinced of the somatic basis of their complaint, many halitophobic patients visit various medical specialists (e.g., dentists, E.N.T, gastroenterologists, etc.) in the hope of finding a cure for their perceived ailment. For example, one study (Seemann et al. 2006) reported that 76% of the halitophobic patients visiting the clinic had received prior treatments for bad breath. Some (36%) had undergone gastroscopies and others (14%) underwent an ENT operation—all without having any detectable signs of bad breath. Only 9% of those patients went through an actual organoleptic evaluation of their breath before they underwent these medical procedures.

12.2   Olfactory Reference Syndrome (ORS)

Halitophobia is considered one manifestation of Olfactory Reference Syndrome (Pryse-Phillips 1971), described as "preoccupation about body odour accompanied by shame, embarrassment, significant distress, avoidance behaviour and social isolation" (Lochner and Stein 2003).

N. Sterer, M. Rosenberg, *Breath Odors*, https://doi.org/10.1007/978-3-030-44731-1_12

Halitophobia has also been considered as a type of monosymptomatic delusion ("delusional halitosis"), alongside parasitosis.

Psychological disorders in which a person is convinced of giving of bodily odors perceived by others have been reported in the literature since the late 1800s. These disorders were termed "Bromidrosiphobia" (Sutton 1919), "Chronic olfactory paranoid syndrome" (Videbech 1966), and "Taijin-kyofusho" (Suzuki et al. 2004).

Pryse-Phillips (1971) noted that in patients suffering from ORS the belief of exuding bodily odors was accompanied by other behaviors such as excessive washing and use of deodorants and perfumes, social avoidance, and multiple medical consultations. Furthermore, ideas of reference were another common feature. Patients believed that people made comments or gestures regarding their bodily odors especially in confined spaces (e.g., trains, buses).

A systematic review (Begum and McKenna 2011) was conducted on ORS case reports based on the following diagnostic criteria:

1. A persistent false belief that one emits a malodorous smell; this belief may encompass a range of insights (i.e., does not have to be delusional).
2. The belief causes clinically significant distress, is time-consuming (i.e., preoccupies the individual for at least 1 h/day) or results in significant impairment of function (whether social, occupational, or other).
3. The belief is not better accounted for by another mental disorder or general medical condition.

This study reported that the mean age of onset for ORS was 21 with 58% of the cases affecting patients less than 20 years old. Low mood was present in 39% and anxiety in 42% of the cases. In 49% of the subjects precipitant events were present, and were mainly (85%) smell-related experiences (remarks or gestures from family members or classmates) accompanied by shame and embarrassment. The smells included feet, underarm, groin, sweat, urine, feces, bad breath, and sexual odors. In 59% of the cases, the patients could not smell the malodor themselves. In 57% the conviction of the perceived odor was fixed or firmly held, whereas in other cases that belief was held with less than full conviction (e.g., admitting that the preoccupation was excessive and unreasonable). Referential ideas in the form of misinterpretations of comments and gestures were common (74%) and were all related to social references. Furthermore, some of the precipitating events may not have been real but rather an early symptom of the disorder.

A study conducted among 421 university students (age 18–24 years) in China reported that the prevalence of ORS was 2.4% and showed no association with gender (Zhou et al. 2018). Interestingly, in that study ORS showed only a weak association with other comorbid disorder symptoms, suggesting that ORS may be considered as a distinct disorder when looking into nonclinical populations.

ORS shows some common features with other psychiatric disorders (Table 12.1). As a result, there is an ongoing debate in the literature regarding the classification of ORS either as a separate disorder or an expansion of another disorder (e.g., a malodor aspect of body dysmorphic disorder).

Unlike common views, which regard ORS as typically chronic, persistent, and tending to worsen over time, the current review (Begum and McKenna 2011) concluded that around two-thirds of the treated cases show improvement or recovery. Of all forms of treatment, the best response was seen with psychotherapy (78%), especially behavioral therapy.

12.3   Back to Halitophobia

Despite the many resembling features stated above there is one key difference between body odors and breath odors. Unlike other bodily odors, a person cannot normally smell his own breath. This physiological fact on the one hand and the relatively large prevalence of breath odors might explain the high proportion of patients that express an exaggerated concern of having a breath odor problem (i.e., Halitophobia). In a study on social phobia conducted in 1997 in

Table 12.1 Similar and dissimilar features of Organoleptic Reference Syndrome (ORS) as compared with other disorders (Begum and McKenna 2011)

Disorder	Organoleptic reference syndrome (ORS) Similar	Dissimilar
Delusional disorder	In most cases, ORS is a delusional belief (complete conviction of emitting malodor).	In some cases ORS has a non-delusional form (good insight, overvalued ideation).
Social phobia	In most cases, ORS patients are concerned about the social implication of emitting malodor (experiencing shame, embarrassment, and anxiety or avoiding social situations).	Social phobia is typically associated with an act (speaking, eating, writing etc.) rather than body odors.
Obsessive compulsive disorder (OCD)	Most cases of ORS show excessive, repetitive compulsive behaviors that are aimed at checking or eliminating the perceived odor.	Only few cases of OCD are delusional, and ideas of reference (how the condition is perceived by others) are much less common.
Body dysmorphic disorder (BDD)	Core belief of a bodily defect that leads to social avoidance. Preoccupation and frequent seeking of medical (nonmental) treatment to alleviate the perceived problem.	The core beliefs, repetitive behaviors and treatment responses may differ. Currently limited to physical defects.
Hypochondriasis	Preoccupation with the body, obsessional thinking, and repetitive behavior (seeking medical diagnosis and treatments).	Hypochondriasis is characterized by a core fear of having a serious disease.

Canada on a population of 1206 subjects (Stein M, unpublished data from a community survey (Stein et al. 2000)), 15.8% worried "a lot" about how their breath smelled, 2.8% had seen a professional about their breath, and 2.7% claimed that their breath concern interfered with their lives (e.g., socially, professionally).

A questionnaire-based study conducted on 4763 participants (Vali et al. 2015) showed that subjective halitosis (i.e., self-reported) was significantly associated with stress, anxiety, and depression. In addition, subjects demonstrating neurotic personality traits were more inclined to this condition. Furthermore, another study conducted on 262 patients treated for confirmed halitosis showed that patients with high scores on the Liebowitz Social Anxiety Scale (LSAS) were still concerned about their oral malodor even following treatment (Zaitsu et al. 2011), suggesting that halitosis and halitophobia can be two separate conditions.

Based on clinical experience and research, halitophobic patients often:

1. Present with a high degree of certainty and conviction that they suffer from bad breath. The descriptions of which are often exaggerated (e.g., very foul smell that can be sensed across the room).

2. Possess a lot of information on the subject of bad breath, often nonscientific in nature.

3. Have had frequent consultations with various medical specialists (e.g., dentists, E.N.T, gastroenterologists, etc.).

4. Practice a high degree of oral hygiene, often obsessively (although they often claim that it does not alleviate the odor).

5. Exhibits a high level of grooming and attention to external appearance.

6. Are sometimes secretive concerning their perceived problem, often confiding in no one over the course of years of distress. They may encounter difficulty in discussing the situation with anyone, including the professional at the consultation. They sometimes break down in tears at the initial consultation. They often bridle and express anger, disbelief, and disappointment when told that their complaint of bad breath has not been verified by the clinical examination.

7. Are often able to somehow carry on with their lives, despite the self-perceived "predicament."

8. Tend to use various evasive methods and avoidance techniques to prevent others from smelling them (e.g., avoiding close encounters of professional or social origin, chewing gum incessantly, and standing downwind during a conversation).

9. Appear to be more concerned by the social implications of their perceived affliction, rather than expressing anxiety that it is a life-threatening medical condition.

Much like ORS patients complaining of other bodily odors, halitophobic patients often report on a precipitating event that is mostly odor related. These may include:

1. Referral comments and remarks by family or friends (e.g., having been told once in the past) a sporadic event that made a lifelong impact (associated with shame and embarrassment).
2. Presence of foul-smelling particles cough up and expelled from the throat (i.e., Tonsilloliths).
3. Having a family member (parent or sibling) with bad breath.

Apart from referral comments and gestures (e.g., rubbing nose, stepping back) that are automatically attributed to breath odors, halitophobic patients also often rely on self-perceived cues such as bad taste and oral dryness as signs for their perceived breath odor. These subjective signs are mostly psychosomatic and are the result of the exaggerated concerns and preoccupation regarding the perceived breath odor problem, rather than real conditions.

Some researchers dealing with the subject of the management of Halitophobic patients have noted that in most cases these patients refuse to accept the fact that their condition is psychological (Yaegaki and Coil 1999). Furthermore, this lack of acceptance and total conviction often leads to confrontation between the doctor and the patient. To avoid these conflicts, it was proposed not to engage in an argument on the objectivity of the complaint, but rather put the emphasis on educating the patient (e.g., oral hygiene instructions). However, research has shown that this type of approach is not successful (Iwu and Akpata 1990), since most of these patients practice good oral hygiene and are looking for a new approach.

In patients who show less conviction in their belief a simple explanation or demonstration (e.g., using Halimeter) may be effective in persuading the patient in the absence of an objective malodor problem. In severe, more delusional cases the resistance would be much higher. Nevertheless, it is the clinician's responsibility not to "skirt the issue" and to inform the patient about his suspected condition. This should be done in an empathetic manner, giving the patient detailed explanation of his condition and recommending psychological consultation when warranted.

References

Begum M, McKenna PJ. Olfactory reference syndrome: a systematic review of the world literature. Psychol Med. 2011;9:1–9.

Iwu CO, Akpata O. Delusional halitosis. Review of the literature and analysis of 32 cases. Br Dent J. 1990;168(7):294–6.

Lochner C, Stein DJ. Olfactory reference syndrome: diagnostic criteria and differential diagnosis. J Postgrad Med. 2003;49(4):328–31.

Pryse-Phillips W. An olfactory reference syndrome. Acta Psychiatr Scand. 1971;47(4):484–509.

Quirynen M, Dadamio J, Van den Velde S, De Smit M, Dekeyser C, Van Tornout M, Vandekerckhove B. Characteristics of 2000 patients who visited a halitosis clinic. J Clin Periodontol. 2009;36(11):970–5.

Rosenberg M, Leib E. Experiences of an Israeli malodor clinic. In: Rosenberg M, editor. Bad breath research perspectives. Tel Aviv: Ramot Publishing—Tel Aviv University; 1997. p. 137–48.

Seemann R, Bizhang M, Djamchidi C, Kage A, Nachnani S. The proportion of pseudo-halitosis patients in a multidisciplinary breath malodour consultation. Int Dent J. 2006;56(2):77–81.

Stein MB, Torgrud LJ, Walker JR. Social phobia symptoms, subtypes, and severity: findings from a community survey. Arch Gen Psychiatry. 2000;57(11):1046–52.

Sutton RL. Bromidrosiphobia. J Am Med Assoc. 1919;72:1267–8.

Suzuki K, Takei N, Iwata Y, Sekine Y, Toyoda T, Nakamura K, Minabe Y, Kawai M, Iyo M, Mori N. Do olfactory reference syndrome and jiko-shu-kyofu (a subtype of taijin-kyofu) share a common entity? Acta Psychiatr Scand. 2004;109(2):150–5. discussion 155.

Vali A, Roohafza H, Keshteli AH, Afghari P, Javad Shirani M, Afshar H, Savabi O, Adibi P. Relationship between subjective halitosis and psychological factors. Int Dent J. 2015;65(3):120–6.

Videbech T. Chronic olfactory paranoid syndromes. A contribution to the psychopathology of the sense of smell. Acta Psychiatr Scand. 1966;42(2):183–213.

Yaegaki K, Coil JM. Clinical dilemmas posed by patients with psychosomatic halitosis. Quintessence Int. 1999;30(5):328–33.

Yaegaki K, Coil JM. Examination, classification, and treatment of halitosis; clinical perspectives. J Can Dent Assoc. 2000;66(5):257–61.

Zaitsu T, Ueno M, Shinada K, Wright FA, Kawaguchi Y. Social anxiety disorder in genuine halitosis patients. Health Qual Life Outcomes. 2011;9:94.

Zhou X, Schneider SC, Cepeda SL, Storch EA. Olfactory reference syndrome symptoms in Chinese university students: phenomenology, associated impairment, and clinical correlates. Compr Psychiatry. 2018;86:91–5.

Oral Malodor Management

13

Contents

The key to successful resolution of a breath odor complaint is its objective diagnosis (for more details, see Chap. 9). First, the physical nature of the complaint has to be verified. Subsequently, the source of the malodor should be determined. Based on these, an appropriate treatment may be suggested and implemented.

Breath odors may arise from a variety of different sources including various systemic and ENT-related conditions (described in Chaps. 5–7). These warrant the referral of the patient to the appropriate physician/specialist. However, in most cases (perhaps 90%), the source of the problem is anaerobic bacterial activity within the oral cavity itself (e.g., tongue, gums, teeth, restorations). Therefore, oral caregivers, i.e., dentists and hygienists should be knowledgeable in this field. They are generally responsible for its treatment.

Successful resolution of a bad breath complaint depends on patient cooperation on two levels: (1) Since self-assessment of oral malodor is mostly unreliable, the patient must enlist the assistance of a close friend or family member to monitor his/her condition. This objective evaluation is not only important for the clinician's diagnosis and follow-up but also imperative for the patient's ability to regain his/her confidence in social situations. (2) Similar to other bacterial-related problems of the oral cavity such as caries and periodontal disease, the long-term successful outcome of oral malodor treatment relies mainly on the patient's ability to maintain good oral hygiene with an emphasis on proper tongue and interdental cleaning.

13.1 Mechanical Therapy

Most of the many different species of bacteria residing in the oral cavity are unable to inhabit any other sites in the human body. Therefore, they are under constant threat of being washed out or swallowed, and their ability to adhere to oral surfaces and form biofilms is imperative to their survival. These oral biofilms are tissue-like structures consisting of cellular and extracellular matrix and are highly resistance to rinsing, washing, detergents, and even antibiotics. This is one reason why mechanical cleaning procedures,

© Springer Nature Switzerland AG 2020

N. Sterer, M. Rosenberg, *Breath Odors*, https://doi.org/10.1007/978-3-030-44731-1_13

such as brushing and cleaning of dental and oral surfaces, are the cornerstone of oral hygiene.

Since the malodor-producing bacteria reside mainly on the posterior area of the tongue dorsum and interdental spaces, areas which are normally inaccessible to regular cleaning, it is not surprising that tooth brushing alone has a very weak short-term effect on oral malodor reduction. The data presented in Table 13.1 show the effect of various oral hygiene procedures on malodor-related parameters.

Table 13.1 Effect of oral hygiene activities on oral malodor and related parameters

Reference (no. of subjects)	Oral hygiene activities	Criteria and malodor parameters	Follow-up duration and outcome
Tonzetich and Ng (1976)	Single activity	VSC (H_2S, GC)	1 h follow-up
($n = 8$)	Brushing:		
	Teeth		29% reduction
	Tongue		74% reduction
	Tongue and teeth		76% reduction
	Eating		83% reduction
Suarez et al. (2000)	Single activity	VSC (H_2S, GC)	8 h follow-up
($n = 8$)	Brushing:		
	Teeth		25% reduction
	Tongue		65% reduction
	Rinsing:		
	3% H_2O_2		90% reduction
	Eating		40% reduction
	No treatment		10% reduction
Seemann et al. (2001a)	Single activity tongue cleaning using:	VSC (Halimeter)	Up to 30 min follow-up
($n = 28$)	Tongue cleaner	>130 ppb included	42% reduction
	Tongue scraper		40% reduction
	Toothbrush		33% reduction
Pedrazzi et al. (2004)	Tongue cleaning (3 times a day for 1 week):	VSC (hand held sulfide monitor)	Follow-up time not stated
($n = 10$)	Tongue scraper		75% reduction
	Toothbrush		40% reduction
Faveri et al. (2006)	3 times a day for 1 week (following professional cleaning):	Odor judge scores (single judge)	8 h follow-up
($n = 19$)	Tooth brushing (TB)	0–3 scale	90% increase (1.1–2.0)
	TB + flossing (Fl)		85% increase (1.1–1.9)
	TB + tongue scraping (TS)		20% increase (1.1–1.3)
	TB + Fl + TS		24% increase (0.9–1.1)
Farrell et al. (2006)	4 times in 24 h	VSC (Halimeter)	3 h follow-up
($n = 26$)	Tooth brushing (NaF)		159 ppb
	Tooth brushing (triclosan)		143 ppb
	Tooth + tongue brushing (triclosan)		126 ppb (significantly better the tooth brushing alone, $p = 0.035$)
Aung et al. (2015)	Twice a day for 1 week:	VSC (Breathtron)	6 h follow-up
($n = 30$)	Tooth brushing (TB)		30% reduction (N.S.)
	Tooth + tongue brushing (TTB)		48% reduction ($p < 0.05$)
	TB + mouthwash (ClO_2)		51% reduction ($p < 0.01$)
	TTB + mouthwash (ClO_2)		72% reduction ($p < 0.01$)
Ileri Keceli et al. (2015)	Twice a day for 2 weeks (following scaling + polishing):	VSC (Halimeter)	2 h follow-up
($n = 69$)	Tooth brushing (TB)		26% reduction ($p < 0.05$)
	Tooth + tongue brushing (TTB)		37% reduction ($p < 0.05$)
Acar et al. (2019)	1 week (following scaling + polishing):	Odor judge scores (single judge)	3 h follow-up
($n = 36$)	Oral hygiene (OH; not specified) without tongue scraping.	0–5 scale	17% increase (1.61–1.89)
	OH + tongue scraping (once a day).		34% decrease (2.28–1.50)

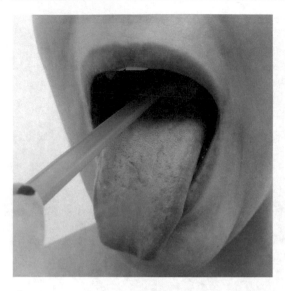

Fig. 13.1 Tongue cleaning using a plastic tongue cleaner

The data presented in this table suggest that tongue cleaning (Fig. 13.1) is the most effective oral hygiene activity in reducing oral malodor and related parameters. Furthermore, it is evident that not all tongue-cleaning methods are equally effective. For instance, cleaning the tongue using a tooth brush appeared to be less effective than using a tongue cleaner designed specifically for this purpose (Pedrazzi et al. 2004; Seemann et al. 2001a). The effect of eating, especially abrasive foods, on malodor reduction was also attributed in part to its tongue-cleaning properties (Suarez et al. 2000). Furthermore, some researchers suggested that in addition to the reduction of malodor-related parameters, the use of a tongue scraper may have a mitigating effect on gingival inflammation (Acar et al. 2019).

It is also important to note that tongue cleaning should be done delicately. The use of sharp or jagged scrapers is not recommended since repeated injuries to the tongue may be harmful.

13.2 Chemical Therapy

Although tongue cleaning seems to be very effective in reducing malodor and malodor-related parameters (e.g., VSC), its effectiveness is relatively short term (less than 2 h). Research done by Quirynen et al. (2004) showed that, although tongue cleaning did reduce tongue coating, it did not reduce the bacterial load on the tongue. In other words, the mechanical cleaning of the tongue appears to affect their food supply (substrate) rather than the bacteria themselves. This was further supported by other researchers who showed that tongue scraping did not have an effect on reducing levels of tongue bacteria (Ademovski et al. 2013). Therefore, in order to achieve long-term efficacy, the use of antimicrobial agents should be considered.

Various chemical agents such as chlorhexidine, cetylpyridinium chloride, essential oils, triclosan, chlorine dioxide, hydrogen peroxide, and zinc have been shown, individually or combined, to be effective in reducing oral malodor (Tables 13.2 and 13.3). The proposed mechanism of action for these agents is mostly antibacterial or antiseptic; however, some of them are able to chemically bind or alter malodor components (e.g., binding of sulfide ions by zinc), rendering them odorless. Therefore, combining different agents with different mechanisms of action (e.g., antibacterial and sulfide binding) may result in a superior outcome.

These antibacterial agents have been incorporated into various delivery systems (e.g., mouthrinses, dentifrices, lozenges) designed to treat oral malodor. However, since oral malodor is generally considered a cosmetic issue for regulatory purposes, many products on the market claim to alleviate oral malodor, yet have relatively little supporting data. In 2003, the American Dental Association (ADA) Council on Scientific Affairs published guidelines for products used in the management of oral malodor regarding the safety and effectiveness of these products (Wozniak 2005). According to these guidelines, safety issues include long-term follow-up (6 months) for adverse effects on soft and hard oral tissues, allergic and toxic effects, and the development of opportunistic and pathogenic organisms. Effectiveness, on the other hand, should be established through well-designed blinded and controlled clinical studies on subjects with oral malodor (odor judge score ≥2, on a 0–5 scale), and the outcome measured by trained and calibrated odor judges (at least two judges).

Table 13.2 Effect of mouthrinses containing various active ingredients on oral malodor and related parameters

Reference (no. of subjects)	Delivery system, application, and active ingredients	Criteria and malodor parameters	Follow-up duration and outcome
Rosenberg et al. (1992)	Mouthrinse (twice for 1 day)	Odor judge scores (single judge)	8–10 h follow-up
(n = 60)	TPM/CPC	0–5 scale	33% reduction (1.5–1)
	0.2% CHX		76% reduction (1.7–0.4)
Kozlovsky et al. (1996)	Mouthrinse (twice a day for 6 weeks)	Odor judge scores (two judges)	≥8 h follow-up
(n = 50)	TPM/CPC	0–5 scale	80% reduction (2.1–0.4)
	EO		70% reduction (2.4–0.7)
Yaegaki and Sanada (1992)	Mouthrinse (single use)	VSC (Halimeter)	3.5 h follow-up
(n = 9)	TPM/CPC	Subjects with ≥75 ppb included	80% reduction
	Control mouthrinse		30% reduction
Bosy et al. (1994)	Mouthrinse (twice a day for 1 week)	Odor judge scores (two judges)	Follow-up time not reported
(n = 101)	0.2% CHX	0–5 scale	64% reduction (2.8–1)
		Subjects with ≥2 included	
Frascella et al. (2000)	Mouthrinse (single use)	Odor judge scores (three judges)	8 h follow-up
(n = 31)	0.1% CD	0–4 intensity scale (−3 to +3 pleasantness scale)	50% reduction (1.2–0.6)
	Control (water)	Subjects with ≤−1 included	9% reduction (1.4–1.3)
Borden et al. (2002)	Mouthrinse (twice a day for 4 weeks)	Odor judge scores (two judges)	4 h follow-up
(n = 95)	EO	0–5 scale	11% reduction (4.1–3.7)
	CPC	Subjects with >2 included	23% reduction (4.2–3.2)
	Placebo		No reduction (3.9–3.9)
	CD/Zn		11% reduction (4–3.6)
Schmidt and Tarbet (1978)	Mouthrinse (single use)	Odor judge scores (three judges)	3 h follow-up
(n = 62)	ZnCl	0–3 scale	37% reduction (1.6–1)
	Control (saline)	Subjects with ≥1 included	14% increase (1.5–1.7)
	No treatment		15% increase (1.6–1.9)
De Boever and Loesche (1995)	Mouthrinse (twice a day for 1 week)	Odor judge scores (single judge)	Follow-up time not reported
(n = 16)	0.12% CHX	0–4 scale	69% reduction (2.9–0.9)
Winkel et al. (2003)	Mouthrinse (twice a day for 2 weeks)	Odor judge scores (single judge)	Follow-up time not reported (morning)
(n = 40)	CHX/CPC/ZnLc (0.05, 0.05, 0.14%)	0–5 scale Subjects with >1 included	46% reduction (2.8–1.5)
	Placebo		7% reduction (2.7–2.5)
Wigger-Alberti et al. (2010)	Mouthrinse (twice a day for 3 weeks)	Odor judge scores (seven judges)	Follow-up time not reported (morning)
(n = 174)	AmF-SnF/ZnLc (0.025, 0.2, 0.12%)	0–5 scale Subjects with >2 included	22% reduction (3.2–2.5)
	CHX/CPC/ZnLc (0.05, 0.05, 0.14%)		26% reduction (3.1–2.3)
	0.12% CHX		27% reduction (3.3–2.4)
	Control (water)		6% reduction (3.2–3)
van Steenberghe et al. (2001)	Mouthrinse (twice a day for 12 days)	Odor judge scores (single judge)	20–30 min follow-up
(n = 12)	0.2% CHX	0–4 scale	78% reduction (1.8–0.4)
	CHX/NaF		89% reduction (1.8–0.2)

Table 13.2 (continued)

Reference (no. of subjects)	Delivery system, application, and active ingredients	Criteria and malodor parameters	Follow-up duration and outcome
	(0.12, 0.05%)		
	CHX/CPC/ZnLc		100% reduction (1.8–0)
	(0.05, 0.05, 0.14%)		
Shinada et al. (2010)	Mouthrinse (twice a day for 7 days)	Odor judge scores (two judges)	Overnight (average 8 h) follow-up
($n = 15$)	0.1% CD	0–5 scale	32% reduction (2.1–1.4)
	Placebo		7% reduction (1.9–1.7)
Rassamee-masmaung et al. (2007)	Mouthrinse (single use)	VSC (Halimeter)	3 h follow-up
($n = 60$)	Herbal	Subjects with ≥80 ppb included	38% reduction
	Placebo		23% reduction
	(twice a day for 2 weeks)		Follow-up time not reported (morning)
	Herbal		60% reduction
	Placebo		26% reduction
Quirynen et al. (2002)	Mouthrinse (twice a day for 7 days)	Odor judge scores (single judge)	20–30 min follow-up
($n = 16$)	0.2% CHX	0–4 scale	88% reduction (1.6–0.2)
	CHX/CPC/ZnLc		81% reduction (1.6–0.3)
	(0.05, 0.05, 0.14%)		
	AmF-SnF		72% reduction (1.8–0.5)
	Placebo		11% reduction (1.8–1.6)
Pitts et al. (1981)	Mouthrinse (single use)	Odor judge scores (five judges)	2 h follow-up
($n = 17$)	EO	1–9 pleasantness scale	9% reduction (6.7–6.1)
	Control (water)		3% increase (6.1–6.3)
Pitts et al. (1983)	Mouthrinse	Odor judge scores (five judges)	3 h follow-up
($n = 30$)	(single use)	1–9 pleasantness scale	
	EO		6% reduction (6.7–6.3)
	Placebo		2% increase (6.6–6.7)
	Control (water)		No reduction (6.7–6.7)
Peruzzo et al. (2007)	Mouthrinse (3 times a day for 4 days)	VSC (Halimeter)	12 h follow-up (morning breath)
($n = 14$)	0.1% CD		12% reduction
	Placebo		112% increase
Carvalho et al. (2004)	Mouthrinse (twice a day for 4 days)	VSC (Halimeter)	12 h follow-up (morning breath)
($n = 12$)	0.2% CHX		70% reduction
	0.12% CHX		63% reduction
	0.03% Triclosan		29% reduction
	EO		24% reduction
	0.05% CPC		14% reduction
	Control (hydro-alc)		21% increase
Wilhelm et al. (2010)	Mouthrinse (single use)	Odor judge scores (eight judges)	4 h follow-up
($n = 42$)	AmF-SnF/ ZnLc	0–5 scale	38% reduction (~2.9–1.8)
	(0.025, 0.2%)	Subjects with ≥2 included	
	CHX/CPC/ZnLc		27% reduction (~2.9–2.1)
	(0.05, 0.05, 0.14%)		
	Control (water)		18% reduction (~3.2–2.6)

(continued)

Table 13.2 (continued)

Reference (no. of subjects)	Delivery system, application, and active ingredients	Criteria and malodor parameters	Follow-up duration and outcome
Ademovski et al. (2013) (*n* = 21)	Mouthrinse (twice a day for 2 weeks)	VSC (Halimeter)	8–12 h follow-up (morning)
	Test MR:		
	ZnAc/CHX/NaF		53% reduction (*p* < 0.01)
	(0.3, 0.025, 0.05%)		
	Test MR + TC		40% reduction (*p* < 0.01)
	Placebo MR		8% reduction (NS)
	Placebo MR + TC		21% reduction (NS)
Dadamio et al. (2013) (*n* = 90)	Mouthrinse (twice a day for 1 week)	Odor judge scores (single judge)	12 h follow-up (morning)
	NaF (0.05%)	0–5 scale	16% reduction (2.4–2.0)
	CHX (0.12%)	Subjects with ≥2 included	39% reduction (2.3–1.4)
	CHX/CPC/ZnLc		53% reduction (2.6–1.2)
	(0.05, 0.5, 0.14%)		
	AmF-SnF		48% reduction (2.7–1.4)
	(0.025%)		
	AmF-SnF/ZnLc		45% reduction (2.4–1.3)
	(0.025, 0.2%)		
Feres et al. (2015) (*n* = 70)	Mouthrinse (twice a day for 3 weeks)	Odor judge scores (three judges)	12 h follow-up (morning)
	Tooth brushing	0–5 scale	59% reduction (3.35–1.37)
	(TB)	Subjects with ≥3 included	
	TB + Mouthrinse		73% reduction (3.36–0.89)
	(CPC 0.075%)		
Ademovski et al. (2013) (*n* = 24)	Mouthrinse (single use)	Odor judge scores (single judge)	12 h follow-up (morning)
	Control (water)	0–5 scale	Compared with control:
	ZnAc/ CHX	Subjects with ≥2 included	B: 47% reduction (2.3–1.2)
	(0.3, 0.025%)		D: 34% reduction (2.3–1.5)
	CHX/CPC/ZnLc		39% reduction (2.3–1.4)
	(0.05, 0.5, 0.14%)		
	ZnCl (0.9%)		30% reduction (2.3–1.6)
	CD (not specified)		43% reduction (2.3–1.3)
Seemann et al. (2016) (*n* = 34)	Mouthrinse (single use)	Odor judge scores (single judge)	12 h follow-up
	Control (water)	0–5 scale	No reduction (2.8–2.8)
	ZnAc/CHX	Subjects with ≥2 included	16% reduction (3.0–2.5)
	(0.3, 0.025%)		
Ademovski et al. (2017) (*n* = 46)	Mouthrinse (twice a day for 6 months)	Odor judge scores (single judge)	Follow-up not specified
	ZnAc/ CHX	0–5 scale	28% reduction (2.8–2.0)
	(0.3, 0.025%)	Subjects with ≥2 included	
	Placebo		7% reduction (2.6–2.4)

TPM two-phase (oil:water) mouthrinse, *CPC* cetylpyridinum chloride, *CHX* chlorhexidine, *EO* essential oils, *CD* chlorine dioxide, *Zn* zinc, *ZnAc* zinc acetate, *ZnCl* zinc chloride, *ZnLc* zinc lactate, *NaF* sodium fluoride, *AmF* amine fluoride, *SnF* stannous fluoride

The most common delivery system for active chemical agents in the treatment of oral malodor is mouthrinse. Table 13.2 shows the results of various clinical trials testing different active ingredients in a mouthrinse formulation on oral malodor and related parameters.

These results show the efficacy of the different active ingredients over varying periods of time ranging from few hours to daylong effects of 10–12 h. It is clear that not all the active ingredients demonstrate the same efficacy in reducing malodor levels. Chlorhexidine (0.2%), which

Table 13.3 Effect of dentifrices and other delivery systems containing various active ingredients on oral malodor and related parameters

Reference (no. of subjects)	Delivery system, application, and active ingredients	Criteria and malodor parameters	Follow-up duration and outcome
Newby et al. (2008)	Dentifrice (single application)	VSC (GC)	1 h follow-up
(n = 16)	0.3% ZnCl (A)	H₂S > 300 ppb included	44% reduction
	0.3% ZnCl (B)		48% reduction
	0.3% Triclosan		26% reduction
	Placebo		24% reduction
Olshan et al. (2000)	Dentifrice (single application)	Odor judge scores (five judges)	1.2 h follow-up
Study 1	EO	1–9 pleasantness scale. Subjects with ≥6 included	23.5% red (7.3–5.6–7.0)
(n = 80)	Control (NaFl)		7.1% red (7.3–6.8–7.2)
Study 2	EO/1% ZnCt		21.3% red (6.5–5.1–6.3)
(n = 90)	Control (NaFl)		7.1% red (6.6–6.1–6.5)
Sharma et al. (1999)	Dentifrice (single application)	Odor judge scores (four judges)	12 h follow-up
(n = 63)	0.3% Triclosan	1–9 pleasantness scale. Subjects with unpleasant breath included	28% reduction (6.6–4.8)
	Control (NaFl)		9% reduction (6.6–6.0)
Waler (1997)	Chewing gum (single application)	VSC (Halimeter)	Immediately following treatment
(n = 11)	2 mg ZnAc		45% reduction
	0.5 mg ZnAc		16% reduction
	Placebo		14% reduction
	Aqueous solution (single application)		
	0.02% ZnCl		45% reduction
	0.2% CHX		7% reduction
	Control (water)		7% reduction
Young et al. (2002)	Lozenges (single application)	VSC (GC)	3 h follow-up
(n = 10)	ZnGl	Cystein challenge	75% reduction
	ZnAc		70% reduction
	ZnCt		No reduction
	ZnAm		70% reduction
Greenstein et al. (1997)	Lozenges (three applications in 24 h)	Odor judge scores (two judges)	2–3 h follow-up
(n = 123)	Oxidizing agent	0–5 scale	50% reduction (1.6–0.8)
	Breath mint		20% reduction (1.6–1.3)
	Chewing gum		17% reduction (1.6–1.3)
	Control		35% reduction (1.6–1.0)
Sterer et al. (2008)	MAT (single application)	Odor judge scores (two judges)	2 h follow-up
(n = 26)	Herbal	0–5 scale	57% reduction (3.4–1.5)
	Placebo		No reduction (3.1–3.4)
Hu et al. (2005)	Dentifrice (twice a day for 3 weeks)	Odor judge scores (four judges)	12 h follow-up (morning breath)
(n = 81)	0.3% Triclosan	1–9 pleasantness scale. Subjects with unpleasant breath included	56% reduction (7.8–3.4)
	Control (NaFl)		9% reduction (7.8–7.1)
Niles et al. (2005)	Dentifrice (twice a day for 1 week)	VSC (GC)	Overnight follow-up (morning breath)
(n = 17)	0.3% Triclosan	>300 ppb included	57% reduction
	Control (NaFl)		10% reduction

(continued)

Table 13.3   (continued)

Reference (no. of subjects)	Delivery system, application, and active ingredients	Criteria and malodor parameters	Follow-up duration and outcome
Nohno et al. (2012)	Tablet (3 times a day for 6 days)	VSC (OralChroma)	1 day follow-up
(n = 14)	CP (3%)		49% reduction
	Placebo		11% increase
Wilhelm et al. (2012)	Tongue gel (twice a day for 1 week)	Odor judge scores (eight judges)	Overnight follow-up
(n = 54)	Tooth brushing (TB) (NaF 0.14%)	0–5 scale	5% reduction (~3.5–3.3)
	TB + tongue cleaning (TC)	Subjects with ≥2 included	3% reduction (~3.3–3.2)
	TB + TC + tongue gel (AmF-SnF/ZnLc)		15% reduction (~3.3–2.8)
	(0.14, 0.5%)		
Sterer et al. (2013)	MAT (twice in 24 h)	Odor judge scores (two judges)	Daylong follow-up (8–10 h)
(n = 40)	Herbal	0–5 scale	32% reduction (2.5–1.7)
	Placebo	Subjects with ≥2 included	11% reduction (2.6–2.3)
	Mouthrinse (EO)		12% reduction (2.4–2.1)
Saad et al. (2016)	Tongue spray (single application)	Odor judge scores (single judge)	6 h follow-up
(n = 21)	Tongue cleaning (TC) + tongue spray (TS; CPC/ZnGl)	0–5 scale	36% reduction (~3.6–2.3)
	(0.09, 0.7%)	Subjects with ≥2 included	
	TC + water		16% reduction (~3.6–3.0)
	TS		5% reduction (~3.6–3.4)
	Water		2% increase (~3.6–3.7)

CHX chlorhexidine, *CP* cystcine protease, *EO* essential oils, *MAT* mucoadhesive tablet, *ZnAc* zinc acetate, *ZnGl* zinc gluconate, *ZnAm* zinc amino chelated, *ZnCl* zinc chloride, *ZnCT* zinc citrate, *ZnLc* zinc lactate, *NaF* sodium fluoride, *AmF* amine fluoride, *SnF* stannous fluoride

appears to be highly effective, is reported to cause many unpleasant side effects (Bosy et al. 1994). Following use of a 0.2% chlorhexidine mouthrinse twice a day for a week 90 out of 101 subjects participating in the study reported some side effect, which included change in the taste of food (60%), burning sensation on the tip of the tongue (26%), staining of the tongue (17%) and teeth (12%), and pain or sloughing of gingival tissue (4%).

The use of an effective mouthrinse (i.e., gargling) has an important part in oral malodor management. Gargling at least once a day should be done on a regular basis in order to control bacterial growth on the tongue dorsum. However, whether regular use of an effective mouthrinse has a cumulative effect is an open question. Whereas, some studies show that repeated use yields better results than a single application

(Kozlovsky et al. 1996; Rassamee-masmaung et al. 2007), others indicate that the effectiveness of the mouthrinse does not improve with a prolonged use (Borden et al. 2002). In any case, this mode of treatment should be applied regularly and constantly.

Some evidence suggest that the regular use of an alcohol-containing mouthrinse might be related to the occurrence of oral and pharyngeal cancer (Winn et al. 1991), possibly attributed to the conversion of alcohol to acetaldehyde by some of the microorganisms in the oral cavity (Shuster et al. 2004). However, since alcohol is not considered an active ingredient and there are many effective mouthrinses available that do not contain alcohol, it might be safer to recommend the use of an alcohol-free mouthrinse.

Due to their relatively short exposure time (typically 1 min), liquid-phase delivery systems (i.e.

mouthrinse) might be limited in efficacy duration. However, some in vitro evidence suggest that formulation modifications such as two-phase solution or the addition of an excipient mucoadhesive agent to the formulation (Jeffet and Sterer 2019) may prolong the bioavailability of its active ingredients.

Other delivery systems for antimicrobial agents, such as dentifrices (tooth paste), lozenges, chewing gums, and mucoadhesive tablets, have also been reported as an effective means to reduce oral malodor (Table 13.3).

Of course, most oral hygiene protocols include the use of toothpaste. At this point, it is important to stress that the detergent in most toothpaste formulations, sodium lauryl sulfate, is anionic and may bind cationic chemical agents (e.g., chlorhexidine, cetylpyridinium chloride) and thus render them inactive. Therefore, it is advisable to keep tooth brushing with toothpaste and gargling with mouthrinse as separate activities.

13.3   Professional Treatment

Some attempts have been made to suggest a treatment need-based classification for oral malodor (Yaegaki and Coil 2000). According to this classification, tongue-related malodor is considered as "physiologic halitosis," thus requiring primarily home care treatments (e.g., improved oral hygiene including regular tongue cleaning combined with mouthrinsing). Conversely, other causes such as periodontal disease and faulty restorations, which require professional treatment, are termed "pathologic halitosis." However, other clinicians (Richter 1996) have suggested that tongue-related malodor is in itself a pathologic condition (i.e. anaerobic bacterial glossitis) that warrants in some cases professional tongue debridment.

The relationship between periodontal disease and oral malodor is not straightforward (Chap. 2). It is likely that both are exacerbated by gingival inflammation brought about by interdental plaque accumulation. Thus, it is not surprising that periodontal treatment, supragingival prophylaxis, and professional teeth cleaning can reduce malodor. Table 13.4 shows a number of studies that looked into the effect of these treatments on oral malodor.

The results of these studies clearly demonstrate the importance of professional treatment in oral malodor management. This is especially true for patients that are unable to maintain good oral hygiene such as the handicapped, elderly, and small children (Adachi et al. 2002; Kara et al. 2006). Professional treatment seems to be particularly beneficial in periodontal

Table 13.4 Effect of professional oral care activities on oral malodor and related parameters

Reference (no. of subjects)	Professional oral care activities	Criteria and malodor parameters	Follow-up duration and outcome
Adachi et al. (2002)	Weekly treatments (scaling and cleaning of teeth, interdental spaces, dentures, and tongue):	VSC (CH$_3$SH, handheld sulfide monitor)	18 months follow-up
($n = 67$)	POHC		Significant difference between groups ($p < 0.05$)
	Control (regular OH)		20 ppb
			55 ppb
Seemann et al. (2001b)	Scaling and polishing compared with tooth brushing and flossing (no tongue cleaning)	VSC (Halimeter)	1 week follow-up
($n = 65$)	PTC		Significant difference between groups ($p < 0.05$)
	TB + Fl		80 ppb
			110 ppb
Seemann et al. (2004)	PTC (scaling and polishing), OH (TB and Fl only)	VSC (Halimeter)	1 month follow-up:
($n = 40$)	No treatment (control)		28% reduction
			No reduction

(continued)

Table 13.4   (continued)

Reference (no. of subjects)	Professional oral care activities	Criteria and malodor parameters	Follow-up duration and outcome
Quirynen et al. (1998)	Test group:	Odor judge scores (single judge	2 months follow-up:
(n = 24)	OSFMD (scaling—root planing, subgingival irrigation, and tongue brushing with 1% CHX gel).	0–3 scale	82% reduction (2.2–0.4)
	Twice a day:	Periodontal patients included	68% reduction (1.9–0.6)
	OH (TB + IDB + TC)		
	Mouthrinse		
	(0.2% CHX)		
	Control:		
	SPT (scaling—root planing)		
	OH (TB + IDB + TC)		
Quirynen et al. (2005)	Combined therapy:	VSC (Halimeter)	6 months follow-up
(n = 45)	OSFMD	Periodontal patients included	65% reduction
	Twice a day:		67% reduction
	OH (TB + IDB + TC)		50% reduction
	Mouthrinse:		
	0.2% CHX		
	0.05% CHX, CPC		
	Placebo		
Tsai et al. (2008)	Sequential treatments	Odor judge scores (single judge, 0–5 scale)	Immediately following treatment:
(n = 25)	Following baseline:	Periodontal patients, malodor scores of ≥2 included	21% reduction (3.8–3.0)
	Tongue scraping (TS)		1 month follow-up:
	2 weeks after TS:		36% reduction (3.8–2.44)
	NSPT (scaling—root planning, faulty restorations removal)		1 month follow-up:
	OH (twice a day)		67% reduction (3.8–1.24)
	1 month after NSPT		
	Twice a day:		
	OH (TB + IDB + TC)		
	Mouthrinse		
	(0.12% CHX, CPC)		
Roldan et al. (2005)	Supragingival prophylaxis	Odor judge scores (single judge, 0–5 scale), malodor scores of ≥1 included	3 months follow-up:
(n = 17)	Twice a day:		50% reduction (2.7–1.4)
	OH (TB + Fl + TC)		
	Mouthrinse		
	(0.05% CHX, CPC, ZnLc)		
Kara et al. (2006)	Scaling	Odor judge scores (single judge, 0–5 scale)	≈3 weeks follow-up:
(n = 150)	OH (tooth and tongue brushing twice a day)	Children (7–12 years old), malodor scores of ≥2 included	85% reduction (3.7–0.5)
Pham et al. (2011)	Periodontitis group:	Odor judge scores (single judge, 0–5 scale), malodor patients included	1 week follow-up:
(n = 218)	NSPT		49% reduction (2.82–1.45)
	TC (once a day)		7% reduction (2.82–2.61)
	Gingivitis group:		12% reduction (2.26–1.98)
	Scaling and polishing		48% reduction (2.33–1.21)
	TC (once a day)		

Table 13.4 (continued)

Reference (no. of subjects)	Professional oral care activities	Criteria and malodor parameters	Follow-up duration and outcome
Soares et al. (2015)	OSFMD compared with SPT:	Odor judge scores (single judge, 0–4 distance scale)	90 days follow-up:
(n = 90)	OSFMD+CHX + TC	Periodontal patients (ppd > 5 mm) included	73% reduction (1.5–0.4)
	OSFMD+CHX		66% reduction (1.8–0.6)
	SPT + TC		90% reduction (2.2–0.2)
	SPT		73% reduction (1.9–0.5)
Dereci et al. (2016)	LSPT (Er,Cr:YSGG)	VSC (Halimeter)	6 months follow-up:
(n = 60)	SPT + LSPT	Periodontal patients included	35% reduction
	SPT		23% reduction
Iatropoulos et al. (2016)	NSPT:	Odor judge scores (single judge, 0–5 scale)	1 week follow-up:
(n = 18)	OH (TB + FL + TC)	Periodontal malodor patients included	15% reduction (3.8–3.2)
	NSPT (scaling and root planning)		25% reduction (3.2–2.3)
Silveira et al. (2017)	OSFMD:	Odor judge scores (single judge, 0–5 scale)	90 days follow-up:
(n = 30)	NSPT	Periodontal patients included	44% reduction (3.8–2.1)
	OSFMD + CHX		62% reduction (3.7–1.4)
	(0.12% mouthrinse twice a day for 2 weeks)		

POHC professional oral health care, *OH* oral hygiene, *PTC* professional tooth cleaning, *TB* tooth brushing, *Fl* flossing, *TC* tongue cleaning, *OSFMD* one-stage full-mouth disinfection, *SPT* standard periodontal therapy, *NSPT* nonsurgical periodontal therapy, *LSPT* laser-supported periodontal therapy, *CPC* cetylpyridinum chloride, *CHX* chlorhexidine, *ZnLc* zinc lactate

patients (Quirynen et al. 2005; Tsai et al. 2008). In fact, some researchers showed that oral hygiene alone (including tongue cleaning) did not eliminate the malodor in periodontal patients (pocket depth >5 mm) when compared with nonsurgical periodontal therapy (Pham et al. 2011).

Interestingly, one-stage full-mouth disinfection yields better results in reducing oral malodor than the standard periodontal therapy (Quirynen et al. 1998). In addition to the standard scaling and root planing (within 24 h), this procedure also includes the use of a disinfecting agent (1% CHX gel) for application within the periodontal pockets and for brushing the tongue. Although it is unclear which of these actions have the most effect on reducing malodor, in periodontal patients and/or those with excessive tongue coating, tongue debridement should be included when performing professional treatment.

References

Acar B, Berker E, Tan Ç, İlarslan YD, Tekçiçek M, Tezcan İ. Effects of oral prophylaxis including tongue cleaning on halitosis and gingival inflammation in gingivitis patients—a randomized controlled clinical trial. Clin Oral Investig. 2019;23(4):1829–36.

Adachi M, Ishihara K, Abe S, Okuda K, Ishikawa T. Effect of professional oral health care on the elderly living in nursing homes. Oral Surg Oral Med Oral Pathol Oral Radiol Endod. 2002;94(2):191–5.

Ademovski SE, Persson GR, Winkel E, Tangerman A, Lingström P, Renvert S. The short-term treatment effects on the microbiota at the dorsum of the tongue in intra-oral halitosis patients—a randomized clinical trial. Clin Oral Investig. 2013;17(2):463–73.

Ademovski SE, Mårtensson C, Persson GR, Renvert S. The long-term effect of a zinc acetate and chlorhexidine diacetate containing mouth rinse on intra-oral halitosis—a randomized clinical trial. J Clin Periodontol. 2017;44(10):1010–9.

Aung EE, Ueno M, Zaitsu T, Furukawa S, Kawaguchi Y. Effectiveness of three oral hygiene regimens on oral malodor reduction: a randomized clinical trial. Trials. 2015;16:31.

Borden LC, Chaves ES, Bowman JP, Fath BM, Hollar GL. The effect of four mouthrinses on oral malodor. Compend Contin Educ Dent. 2002;23(6):531–6, 538, 540 passim; quiz 548.

Bosy A, Kulkarni GV, Rosenberg M, McCulloch CA. Relationship of oral malodor to periodontitis: evidence of independence in discrete subpopulations. J Periodontol. 1994;65(1):37–46.

Carvalho MD, Tabchoury CM, Cury JA, Toledo S, Nogueira-Filho GR. Impact of mouthrinses on morning bad breath in healthy subjects. J Clin Periodontol. 2004;31(2):85–90.

Dadamio J, Van Tournout M, Teughels W, Dekeyser C, Coucke W, Quirynen M. Efficacy of different mouthrinse formulations in reducing oral malodour: a randomized clinical trial. J Clin Periodontol. 2013;40(5):505–13.

De Boever EH, Loesche WJ. Assessing the contribution of anaerobic microflora of the tongue to oral malodor. J Am Dent Assoc. 1995;126(10):1384–93.

Dereci Ö, Hatipoğlu M, Sindel A, Tozoğlu S, Üstün K. The efficacy of Er,Cr:YSGG laser supported periodontal therapy on the reduction of periodontal disease related oral malodor: a randomized clinical study. Head Face Med. 2016;12(1):20.

Farrell S, Baker RA, Somogyi-Mann M, Witt JJ, Gerlach RW. Oral malodor reduction by a combination of chemotherapeutical and mechanical treatments. Clin Oral Investig. 2006;10(2):157–63.

Faveri M, Hayacibara MF, Pupio GC, Cury JA, Tsuzuki CO, Hayacibara RM. A cross-over study on the effect of various therapeutic approaches to morning breath odour. J Clin Periodontol. 2006;33(8):555–60.

Feres M, Figueiredo LC, Faveri M, Guerra MC, Mateo LR, Stewart B, Williams M, Panagakos F. The efficacy of two oral hygiene regimens in reducing oral malodour: a randomised clinical trial. Int Dent J. 2015;65(6):292–302.

Frascella J, Gilbert RD, Fernandez P, Hendler J. Efficacy of a chlorine dioxide-containing mouthrinse in oral malodor. Compend Contin Educ Dent. 2000;21(3):241–4, 246, 248 passim; quiz 256.

Greenstein RB, Goldberg S, Marku-Cohen S, Sterer N, Rosenberg M. Reduction of oral malodor by oxidizing lozenges. J Periodontol. 1997;68(12):1176–81.

Hu D, Zhang YP, Petrone M, Volpe AR, Devizio W, Giniger M. Clinical effectiveness of a triclosan/copolymer/sodium fluoride dentifrice in controlling oral malodor: a 3-week clinical trial. Oral Dis. 2005;11(Suppl 1):51–3.

Iatropoulos A, Panis V, Mela E, Stefaniotis T, Madianos PN, Papaioannou W. Changes of volatile sulphur compounds during therapy of a case series of patients with chronic periodontitis and halitosis. J Clin Periodontol. 2016;43(4):359–65.

Ileri Keceli T, Gulmez D, Dolgun A, Tekcicek M. The relationship between tongue brushing and halitosis in children: a randomized controlled trial. Oral Dis. 2015;21(1):66–73.

Jeffet U, Sterer N. Effect of mucoadhesive agent HEC on herbal extracts retention and VSC producing bacteria reduction in an experimental oral biofilm. J Breath Res. 2019;13(2):026004.

Kara C, Tezel A, Orbak R. Effect of oral hygiene instruction and scaling on oral malodour in a population of Turkish children with gingival inflammation. Int J Paediatr Dent. 2006;16(6):399–404.

Kozlovsky A, Goldberg S, Natour I, Rogatky-Gat A, Gelernter I, Rosenberg M. Efficacy of a 2-phase oil: water mouthrinse in controlling oral malodor, gingivitis, and plaque. J Periodontol. 1996;67(6):577–82.

Newby EE, Hickling JM, Hughes FJ, Proskin HM, Bosma MP. Control of oral malodour by dentifrices measured by gas chromatography. Arch Oral Biol. 2008;53(Suppl 1):S19–25.

Niles HP, Hunter C, Vazquez J, Williams MI, Cummins D. The clinical comparison of a triclosan/copolymer/fluoride dentifrice vs a breath-freshening dentifrice in reducing breath odor overnight: a crossover study. Oral Dis. 2005;11(Suppl 1):54–6.

Nohno K, Yamaga T, Kaneko N, Miyazaki H. Tablets containing a cysteine protease, actinidine, reduce oral malodor: a crossover study. J Breath Res. 2012;6(1):017107.

Olshan AM, Kohut BE, Vincent JW, Borden LC, Delgado N, Qaqish J, Sharma NC, McGuire JA. Clinical effectiveness of essential oil-containing dentifrices in controlling oral malodor. Am J Dent. 2000;13(Spec No):18C–22C.

Pedrazzi V, Sato S, de Mattos MG, Lara EH, Panzeri H. Tongue-cleaning methods: a comparative clinical trial employing a toothbrush and a tongue scraper. J Periodontol. 2004;75(7):1009–12.

Peruzzo DC, Jandiroba PF, Nogueira Filho Gda R. Use of 0.1% chlorine dioxide to inhibit the formation of morning volatile sulphur compounds (VSC). Braz Oral Res. 2007;21(1):70–4.

Pham TA, Ueno M, Zaitsu T, Takehara S, Shinada K, Lam PH, Kawaguchi Y. Clinical trial of oral malodor treatment in patients with periodontal diseases. J Periodontal Res. 2011;46(6):722–9.

Pitts G, Pianotti R, Feary TW, McGuiness J, Masurat T. The in vivo effects of an antiseptic mouthwash on odor-producing microorganisms. J Dent Res. 1981;60(11):1891–6.

Pitts G, Brogdon C, Hu L, Masurat T, Pianotti R, Schumann P. Mechanism of action of an antiseptic, anti-odor mouthwash. J Dent Res. 1983;62(6):738–42.

Quirynen M, Mongardini C, van Steenberghe D. The effect of a 1-stage full-mouth disinfection on oral malodor and microbial colonization of the tongue in periodontitis. A pilot study. J Periodontol. 1998;69(3):374–82.

Quirynen M, Avontroodt P, Soers C, Zhao H, Pauwels M, Coucke W, van Steenberghe D. The efficacy of amine fluoride/stannous fluoride in the suppression of morning breath odour. J Clin Periodontol. 2002;29(10):944–54.

Quirynen M, Avontroodt P, Soers C, Zhao H, Pauwels M, van Steenberghe D. Impact of tongue cleansers on microbial load and taste. J Clin Periodontol. 2004;31(7):506–10.

Quirynen M, Zhao H, Soers C, Dekeyser C, Pauwels M, Coucke W, Steenberghe D. The impact of periodontal therapy and the adjunctive effect of antiseptics on breath odor-related outcome variables: a double-blind randomized study. J Periodontol. 2005;76(5):705–12.

Rassamee-masmaung S, Sirikulsathean A, Amornchat C, Hirunrat K, Rojanapanthu P, Gritsanapan W. Effects of herbal mouthwash containing the pericarp extract of Garcinia mangostana L on halitosis, plaque and papillary bleeding index. J Int Acad Periodontol. 2007;9(1):19–25.

Richter JL. Diagnosis and treatment of halitosis. Compend Contin Educ Dent. 1996;17(4):370–2, 374–6 passim; quiz 388.

Roldan S, Herrera D, O'Connor A, Gonzalez I, Sanz M. A combined therapeutic approach to manage oral halitosis: a 3-month prospective case series. J Periodontol. 2005;76(6):1025–33.

Rosenberg M, Gelernter I, Barki M, Bar-Ness R. Day-long reduction of oral malodor by a two-phase oil:water mouthrinse as compared to chlorhexidine and placebo rinses. J Periodontol. 1992;63(1):39–43.

Saad S, Gomez-Pereira P, Hewett K, Horstman P, Patel J, Greenman J. Daily reduction of oral malodor with the use of a sonic tongue brush combined with an antibacterial tongue spray in a randomized cross-over clinical investigation. J Breath Res. 2016;10(1):016013.

Schmidt NF, Tarbet WJ. The effect of oral rinses on organoleptic mouth odor ratings and levels of volatile sulfur compounds. Oral Surg Oral Med Oral Pathol. 1978;45(6):876–83.

Seemann R, Kison A, Bizhang M, Zimmer S. Effectiveness of mechanical tongue cleaning on oral levels of volatile sulfur compounds. J Am Dent Assoc. 2001a;132(9):1263–7. quiz 1318.

Seemann R, Passek G, Zimmer S, Roulet JF. The effect of an oral hygiene program on oral levels of volatile sulfur compounds (VSC). J Clin Dent. 2001b;12(4):104–7.

Seemann R, Passek G, Bizhang M, Zimmer S. Reduction of oral levels of volatile sulfur compounds (VSC) by professional toothcleaning and oral hygiene instruction in non-halitosis patients. Oral Health Prev Dent. 2004;2(4):397–401.

Seemann R, Filippi A, Michaelis S, Lauterbach S, John HD, Huismann J. Duration of effect of the mouthwash CB12 for the treatment of intra-oral halitosis: a double-blind, randomised, controlled trial. J Breath Res. 2016;10(3):036002.

Sharma NC, Galustians HJ, Qaquish J, Galustians A, Rustogi KN, Petrone ME, Chaknis P, Garcia L, Volpe AR, Proskin HM. The clinical effectiveness of a dentifrice containing triclosan and a copolymer for controlling breath odor measured organoleptically twelve hours after toothbrushing. J Clin Dent. 1999;10(4):131–4.

Shinada K, Ueno M, Konishi C, Takehara S, Yokoyama S, Zaitsu T, Ohnuki M, Wright FA, Kawaguchi Y. Effects of a mouthwash with chlorine dioxide on oral malodor and salivary bacteria: a randomized placebo-controlled 7-day trial. Trials. 2010;11:14.

Shuster A, Osherov N, Rosenberg M. Alcohol-mediated haemolysis in yeast. Yeast. 2004;21(16):1335–42.

Silveira JO, Costa FO, Oliveira PAD, Dutra BC, Cortelli SC, Cortelli JR, Cota LOM, Oliveira AMSD. Effect of non-surgical periodontal treatment by full-mouth disinfection or scaling and root planing per quadrant in halitosis—a randomized controlled clinical trial. Clin Oral Investig. 2017;21(5):1545–52.

Soares LG, Castagna L, Weyne SC, Silva DG, Falabella MEV, Tinoco EMB. Effectiveness of full- and partial-mouth disinfection on halitosis in periodontal patients. J Oral Sci. 2015;57(1):1–6.

Sterer N, Nuas S, Mizrahi B, Goldenberg C, Weiss EI, Domb A, Davidi MP. Oral malodor reduction by a palatal mucoadhesive tablet containing herbal formulation. J Dent. 2008;36(7):535–9.

Sterer N, Ovadia O, Weiss EI, Perez Davidi M. Day-long reduction of oral malodor by a palatal mucoadhesive tablet containing herbal formulation. J Breath Res. 2013;7(2):026004.

Suarez FL, Furne JK, Springfield J, Levitt MD. Morning breath odor: influence of treatments on sulfur gases. J Dent Res. 2000;79(10):1773–7.

Tonzetich J, Ng SK. Reduction of malodor by oral cleansing procedures. Oral Surg Oral Med Oral Pathol. 1976;42(2):172–81.

Tsai CC, Chou HH, Wu TL, Yang YH, Ho KY, Wu YM, Ho YP. The levels of volatile sulfur compounds in mouth air from patients with chronic periodontitis. J Periodontal Res. 2008;43(2):186–93.

van Steenberghe D, Avontroodt P, Peeters W, Pauwels M, Coucke W, Lijnen A, Quirynen M. Effect of different mouthrinses on morning breath. J Periodontol. 2001;72(9):1183–91.

Waler SM. The effect of zinc-containing chewing gum on volatile sulfur-containing compounds in the oral cavity. Acta Odontol Scand. 1997;55(3):198–200.

Wigger-Alberti W, Gysen K, Axmann EM, Wilhelm KP. Efficacy of a new mouthrinse formulation on the reduction of oral malodour in vivo. A randomized, double-blind, placebo-controlled, 3 week clinical study. J Breath Res. 2010;4:017102.

Wilhelm D, Gysen K, Himmelmann A, Krause C, Wilhelm KP. Short-term effect of a new mouthrinse formulation on oral malodour after single use in vivo: a comparative, randomized, single-blind, parallel-group clinical study. J Breath Res. 2010;4(3):036002.

Wilhelm D, Himmelmann A, Axmann EM, Wilhelm KP. Clinical efficacy of a new tooth and tongue gel applied with a tongue cleaner in reducing oral halitosis. Quintessence Int. 2012;43(8):709–18.

Winkel EG, Roldan S, Van Winkelhoff AJ, Herrera D, Sanz M. Clinical effects of a new mouthrinse containing chlorhexidine, cetylpyridinium chloride and zinc-lactate on oral halitosis. A dual-center, double-blind placebo-controlled study. J Clin Periodontol. 2003;30(4):300–6.

Winn DM, Blot WJ, McLaughlin JK, Austin DF, Greenberg RS, Preston-Martin S, Schoenberg JB, Fraumeni JF Jr. Mouthwash use and oral conditions in the risk of oral and pharyngeal cancer. Cancer Res. 1991;51(11):3044–7.

Wozniak WT. The ADA guidelines on oral malodor products. Oral Dis. 2005;11(Suppl 1):7–9.

Yaegaki K, Coil JM. Examination, classification, and treatment of halitosis; clinical perspectives. J Can Dent Assoc. 2000;66(5):257–61.

Yaegaki K, Sanada K. Effects of a two-phase oil-water mouthwash on halitosis. Clin Prev Dent. 1992;14(1):5–9.

Young A, Jonski G, Rolla G. The oral anti-volatile sulphur compound effects of zinc salts and their stability constants. Eur J Oral Sci. 2002;110(1):31–4.

History of Breath Odors

14

Contents

14.1   Culture and Folklore

Breath odors are an age-old worldwide problem, and over the centuries different cultures have developed different folk remedies. In Thailand, sufferers chew the peels of oversize guavas. Iraqis keep cloves between their teeth. Italians chew parsley. Indians chew fennel seeds. Brazilians cite cinnamon as a folk remedy. Indeed, many plant extracts contain antibacterial molecules. These molecules are often oily and aromatic, and can be extracted as part of the "essential oil" fraction. Essential oils are used in mouthrinses, toothpastes, and chewing gums, sometimes for their antibacterial effect, and sometimes for their aroma. Essential oil compounds that inhibit oral microorganisms include eugenol from clove, thymol from thyme, and eucalyptol from eucalyptus. Chinese imbibe crushed eggshells in rice wine, but will also eat a grapefruit for alcohol breath, and for garlic odor, persimmon, or red dates. Traditional Chinese pharmacies, offer a concoction of bark, leaves, and other dried items for relief of too much "heatiness" (yang) which they believe is a major cause of bad breath. Finally, almost all of us believe in the mouth-freshening potential of mint (although actually, most types of mint are not very effective).

Bad breath is discussed at length in the Jewish Talmud, as well as by Egyptian, Greek, and Roman writers. The most ancient recorded remedy for bad breath may date back to Chap. 14, the book of Genesis. Joseph, having been thrown into a pit by his spiteful brothers, is taken to Egypt by a caravan of Ishmaelites. The Bible tells us that the camels bore spices, balm, and ladanum. Because of later writings in the Talmud, we can deduce that ladanum might refer to gum mastic, the resin of the *Pistacia lentiscus*, a small tree that flourishes in the Mediterranean basin (Fig. 14.1). It was produced since Biblical times by making incisions in the bark of the tree during summer months and collecting the resin drops. Gum mastic has been chewed around the Mediterranean for thousands of years, and is still farmed on the Greek island of Chios, off the shore of Turkey. Quite remarkably, this gum has antibacterial properties, and has been used for various medicinal and dental purposes over the centuries.

© Springer Nature Switzerland AG 2020
N. Sterer, M. Rosenberg, *Breath Odors*, https://doi.org/10.1007/978-3-030-44731-1_14

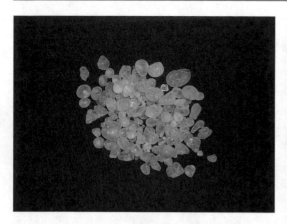

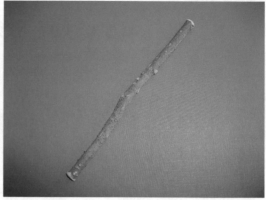

Fig. 14.1 Mastic gum; resin pieces from the *Pestacia lentiscus* tree

Fig. 14.2 Siwak; a stick used by muslims to clean the mouth

Bad breath remedies have been prevalent since the earliest recorded times. The Ebers papyrus, over 3500 years old (University of Leipzig library), describes aromatic concoctions proposed to counter dental ailments, including swollen gums. Some 2000 years ago, the Roman perfume entrepreneur *Cosmo* supposedly sold breath freshening pastilles to his fellow friends and countrymen. His competitors questioned their efficacy.

Ancient Judaism regarded bad breath as a severe infliction, akin to having lost a limb, or suffering from leprosy. According to the Talmud (dating back over 1500 years), priests were not allowed to carry out holy duties in the Temple if they had bad breath (Shifman et al. 2002). According to Jewish law, a man who marries a woman and subsequently discovers that she has bad breath, can summarily divorce her without even fulfilling the terms of the marriage contract (*ketuba*). This differs from medieval Welsh law, in which a wife was able to divorce her husband on the grounds of oral malodor (Paul Meara, University of Wales Swansea, personal communication).

According to the Jewish Talmud, working with flax predisposes to bad breath. In ancient times, flax fibers were wet by saliva in order to spin them into a finer yarn. According to the Talmud this activity damages the woman's lips and causes bad breath, and therefore a husband may not compel his wife to spin flax (Nahum Ben Yehuda, Bar Ilan University, personal communication).

Specific vegetables are mentioned in the Talmud as bad breath risks, particularly raw peas and extensive consumption of lentils. The Talmud suggests a variety of remedies aromatic spices, including ginger and cinnamon, as oral fresheners. Another recommended remedy is the mastic chewing gum described above. The Talmud states that while frivolous chewing of mastic is forbidden on the Sabbath, it is allowed as a cure for bad breath.

Islam also deals at length with bad breath and oral hygiene. There is the famous story that the prophet Muhammad once asked someone to leave the mosque because of his bad breath. Islam stresses the importance of hygiene and good smells. A case in point is the *siwak* (sometimes spelled sewak or miswak), a short stick which is regarded by Moslems as a holy instrument (Fig. 14.2). By wetting and chewing or pounding on one of the ends, a kind of toothbrush is formed which can be used to clean both teeth and soft tissue. Siwaks are made from the aerial roots of certain trees and may contain antibacterial agents. Modern mint-flavored siwaks are also available.

Bad breath is usually considered taboo in Islam, as it is in Judaism. One exception is bad breath due to fasting during the Ramadan, which according to Islamic teaching is considered by Allah to be more esteemed than the smell of roses.

During medieval times in the ninth century, the first medical school was founded in Salerno, Italy. The Salerno Medical School translated and preserved the medical knowledge accumulated from the Greek–Latin, Jewish and Arabic cultures. Its scholars have written many important manuscripts referring also to dental care and oral hygiene. Trotula De Ruggiero, considered the most famous female practitioner of the school suggested an oral hygiene regimen that included mechanical tooth cleaning and the use of various plants and minerals that are still considered beneficial today such as date (*Phoenix dactylifera*), fennel (Foeniculum), marrow (Cucurbita), pepper (Piper nigrum L.), parsley (Petroselinum), Armenian bole (Bolus armenus), calcium carbonate, and sodium carbonate (Bifulco et al. 2016)

14.2   Early Scientific and Medical Literature

In the late eighteenth century, Dr. Joseph W. Howe wrote a medical text on bad breath, which was published in four editions from 1874 to 1898 ("The Breath and the Diseases which give it a fetid odor with directions for treatment"; D. Appleton and company, 1898). Dr. Howe was inter alia Professor of Clinical Surgery at Bellevue Hospital Medical College.

According to Dr. Howe, bad breath is liable to occur at all periods of life, and is more common among menfolk. "*Yet how few of the afflicted persons detect the cause of their isolation, or recognize the barrier which effectually prevents the approach of those near and dear to them!*" He wrote of the difficulty in telling someone that they suffer from bad breath. "*With the best intentions in the world, we rarely whisper a word of their disorder or suggest a source of relief. This false kindness—this demoralizing weakness—is universal.*"

Dr. Howe clearly linked bad breath to the oral cavity. "*When the teeth and mucous membrane of the mouth are kept clean…the offensive odor of the breath will disappear.*"

He also alerted parents to malodor due to nasal foreign bodies in children. "*Children of tender years frequently insert peas, beans, and foreign substances into the nasal cavities, which enlarge by the absorption of moisture, and, by and increase of pressure, cause great irritation. Peas and beans have been known to sprout in the nasal cavities after having remained there several days, giving rise to serious inflammation of the mucous membrane and spongy bones. The discharge takes place generally from the nostril in which the foreign body is located.*"

Some of the oral remedies recommended by Dr. Howe, such as carbolic acid (phenol), are toxic and would likely not be condoned in this day and age. Other active ingredients which he recommended include powdered cinnamon, cardamom, oil of nutmeg, rhubarb, myrrh and oil of peppermint, charcoal cake, powdered coriander, sweet-flag (hallucinogenic at high concentrations), and leaves of partridge-berry (*Gaultheria procumbens*). For cigarette smokers, he recommended small pieces of cascarilla or cinnamon bark. For tongue coating (which he considered related to digestive disorders), he recommended scraping the tongue, and washing the mouth with a solution of myrrh tincture and lavender water.

Another worthy reference from the nineteenth century is the review by D.C. Hawxhurst (1873). He was keenly aware of the importance of post-nasal drip ("catarrh") as a major cause of bad breath and wrote about the importance of tonsilloliths:

> In the fauces there sometimes occur little nodular bodies, made up of cheese-like matter, which constitutes the source of a peculiar fetor.

He also alerted his colleagues to odors resulting from diet:

> The diet too should receive attention. …Known polluters of the breath, such as beer, wine, sourkrout, and hard cider, may easily be entirely avoided.

Hawxhurst was keenly aware and also cautioned his dentist colleagues to avail themselves of the kindly offices of "some trustworthy friend," to let them know if they suffered from bad breath.

14.3   Modern History

During the first half of the twentieth century, in the 1930s and 1940s dental researchers such as Glenn F. Sulser and Leonard S. Fosdick from the Northwestern University Dental School in Chicago, began studying the microbial and bio-chemical aspects of oral malodor production using salivary incubation assays. They were the first researchers to demonstrate that oral malodor production comes from the anaerobic microbial degradation of proteins into foul smelling by-products (Berg et al. 1946; Fosdick and Piez 1953). They discovered the relationship between salivary putrefaction and periodontal disease (Berg et al. 1947), and were the first to try and quantify oral malodor instrumentally using the Osmoscope (Brening et al. 1939; Fig. 14.3).

In 1933, an American dentist named G.L. Grapp published a paper summarizing a study of 500 patients (Grapp 1933). He con-cluded that most bad breath comes from the back of the tongue. He found that the tongues of 90% of those he checked had a visible coating. Grapp showed that the posterior (back) two-thirds of the tongue were responsible for the odor by wiping that area with gauze, and then smelling it. Grapp suggested that bad breath arose from insufficient chewing of foods by modern man. He also designed a tongue cleaner and showed that breath improves when the very back of the tongue is cleaned. Actually, tongue cleaning has been prac-ticed in India for hundreds, if not thousands, of years (it is taught in their ancient Ayurveda medi-cine). Furthermore, tongue cleaners were also used in Europe since the mid nineteenth century. A collection of these antique tongue cleaners is on display at the British Dental Association museum (64 WIMPOLE ST., LONDON).

In the 1960s, Joseph Tonzetich from the University of British Columbia in Canada dem-onstrated the role of volatile sulfide compounds, especially hydrogen sulfide and methyl mercap-tan as important components of oral malodor (Tonzetich et al. 1967). Dr. Tonzetich pioneered the use of gas chromatography combined with a flame photometric detector in breath analysis (Tonzetich 1971) and is widely considered the modern day pioneer of the entire field.

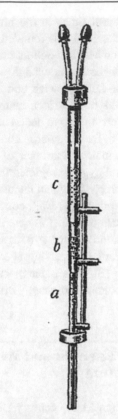

Type B metal osmo-scope. For use with air or liquid dilution method of threshold odour determinations

Fig. 14.3 The Fair–Wells osmoscopes 1935 (with per-mission from IOPscience)

In the early 1970s, Thomas F McNamara showed the role of Gram-negative rather than Gram-positive oral bacteria in malodor produc-tion (McNamara et al. 1972). McNamara also demonstrated the inhibitory effect of glucose and acidic pH on the process of malodor production.

References

Berg M, Burrill DY, Fosdick LS. Chemical studies in peri-odontal disease III: putrefaction of salivary proteins. J Dent Res. 1946;25:231–46.

Berg M, Burrill DY, Fosdick LS. Chemical studies in periodontal disease; putrefaction rate as index of peri-odontal disease. J Dent Res. 1947;26(1):67–71.

Bifulco M, Amato M, Gangemi G, Marasco M, Caggiano M, Amato A, Pisanti S. Dental care and dentistry practice in the Medieval Medical School of Salerno. Br Dent J. 2016;221(2):87–9.

Brening RH, Sulser GF, Fosdick LS. The determination of halitosis by the use of the osmoscope and the cryoscopic method. J Dent Res. 1939;18(2):127–32.

Fosdick LS, Piez KA. Chemical studies in periodontal disease. X. Paper chromatographic investigation of the putrefaction associated with periodontitis. J Dent Res. 1953;32(1):87–100.

Grapp GL. Fetor oris (halitosis): a medical and dental responsibility. Northwest Med. 1933;32:375–80.

Hawxhurst D. Offensive breath. Dent Reg. 1873;27:105–10.

McNamara TF, Alexander JF, Lee M. The role of microorganisms in the production of oral malodor. Oral Surg Oral Med Oral Pathol. 1972;34(1):41–8.

Shifman A, Orenbuch S, Rosenberg M. Bad breath—a major disability according to the Talmud. Isr Med Assoc J. 2002;4(10):843–5.

Tonzetich J. Direct gas chromatographic analysis of sulphur compounds in mouth air in man. Arch Oral Biol. 1971;16(6):587–97.

Tonzetich J, Eigen E, King WJ, Weiss S. Volatility as a factor in the inability of certain amines and indole to increase the odour of saliva. Arch Oral Biol. 1967;12(10):1167–75.

Future Prospects

15

Content

A growing body of knowledge has accumulated over the last 60 years in the field of breath odor research. This has enabled researchers and clinicians to continually build on the scientific findings, devising better means for understanding, diagnosing, and managing this common human condition. However, some important questions regarding this issue are still left open and require further investigation.

It is clear that breath odors are primarily the result of bacterial activity within the oral cavity. However, many of these bacteria are prevalent in the adult population and are not always linked to disease. Therefore, it is safe to assume that other factors (oral conditions, salivary composition, the immune system, etc.) play a role in promoting malodor production. Identifying these promoting factors (e.g., genetic and environmental factors), will give us a better understanding of this condition and will help us recognize possible risk factors.

To this day there is not one reliable instrumental method to measure breath odor. In fact, the gold standard in this field remains the human nose. Using odor judges to evaluate and rate the malodor presents many problems especially in clinical settings. The reason that most currently available instrumental methods show only a moderate concurrence with the human nose (i.e., Pearson r values of around 0.6) derives most probably from the fact that most of these instruments rely on the measurement of VSCs which may represent only some of the gases contributing to breath odors. There have been a few attempts to develop a sensor array (also known as "electronic nose") capable of measuring several different chemical compounds to measure breath, so far without success.

Our inability to sense our own breath odor presents major problems regarding self-diagnosis and post treatments satisfaction. This also prevents people from seeking diagnosis and may create debilitating psychological issues. Therefore, devising a personalize breath analyzer is a matter of top priority in this field. We envision that in the future, highly sensitive odor chips will be available, that can be incorporated in mobile phones, enabling practically everyone to check their breath "on the go."

Given the bacterial nature of this condition, it is not surprising that most treatment approaches rely on antiseptic compounds as an important tool. However, most of these antiseptics commonly found in oral rinses are nonspecific and kill all types of oral bacteria indiscriminately.

Some attempts have been made to utilize a more selective approach, e.g., the in vitro exposure of bacterial samples to various wavelengths of light, either with or without using photosensitizing agents (Soukos et al. 2005) showed this technique to be potentially selective against anaerobic oral bacteria, most likely due to the phototoxic effect that is mediated by the formation of reactive oxygen species (ROS). Furthermore, exposure to blue light has dramatically reduced malodor production by oral bacteria mixtures concomitant with reduction in the proportion of anaerobic Gram-negative bacteria (Sterer and Feuerstein 2005). The addition of a photosensitizing agent was shown to improve the antibacterial and antimalodor phototoxic effect both in vitro (Jeffet et al. 2016) and in vivo (Lopes et al. 2016). However, the effectiveness of photodynamic therapy in breath odors is still an open question (Kellesarian et al. 2017).

Other approaches using nonchemical selective active ingredients such as various herbal medicinals or probiotics were also reported to be effective against anaerobic oral bacteria (Burton et al. 2006; Sterer and Rubinstein 2006). Furthermore, applying these active ingredients using a sustained release delivery system showed them to be effective in reducing oral malodor in human subjects (Sterer et al. 2008).

Major projects carried out over the last decade such as the genome mapping of oral bacteria (for more details, see Chap. 3) and deep sequencing of microbiome has opened the doors for a better understanding of the microbial ecology underlying breath odors as well as supplying an opportunity for personalizing treatments. Research has demonstrated that machine learning-based classification of breath odors that rely on the microbiome of saliva samples is possible (Nakano et al. 2014) and that specific enzymes involved in the malodor production process can be targeted (Kandalam et al. 2018).

These and other questions are under study by many researchers around the world currently involved in this ever-growing field of breath odor research.

References

Burton JP, Chilcott CN, Moore CJ, Speiser G, Tagg JR. A preliminary study of the effect of probiotic Streptococcus salivarius K12 on oral malodour parameters. J Appl Microbiol. 2006;100(4):754–64.

Jeffet U, Nasrallah R, Sterer N. Effect of red dyes on blue light phototoxicity against VSC producing bacteria in an experimental oral biofilm. J Breath Res. 2016;10(4):046011.

Kandalam U, Ledra N, Laubach H, Venkatachalam KV. Inhibition of methionine gamma lyase deaminase and the growth of Porphyromonas gingivalis: a therapeutic target for halitosis/periodontitis. Arch Oral Biol. 2018;90:27–32.

Kellesarian SV, Malignaggi VR, Al-Kheraif AA, Al-Askar M, Yunker M, Javed F. Effect of antimicrobial photodynamic therapy and laser alone as adjunct to mechanical debridement in the management of halitosis: a systematic review. Quintessence Int. 2017;48(7):575–83.

Lopes RG, da Mota AC, Soares C, Tarzia O, Deana AM, Prates RA, França CM, Fernandes KP, Ferrari RA, Bussadori SK. Immediate results of photodynamic therapy for the treatment of halitosis in adolescents: a randomized, controlled, clinical trial. Lasers Med Sci. 2016;31(1):41–7.

Nakano Y, Takeshita T, Kamio N, Shiota S, Shibata Y, Suzuki N, Yoneda M, Hirofuji T, Yamashita Y. Supervised machine learning-based classification of oral malodor based on the microbiota in saliva samples. Artif Intell Med. 2014;60(2):97–101.

Soukos NS, Som S, Abernethy AD, Ruggiero K, Dunham J, Lee C, Doukas AG, Goodson JM. Phototargeting oral black-pigmented bacteria. Antimicrob Agents Chemother. 2005;49(4):1391–6.

Sterer N, Feuerstein O. Effect of visible light on malodour production by mixed oral microflora. J Med Microbiol. 2005;54(Pt 12):1225–9.

Sterer N, Rubinstein Y. Effect of various natural medicinals on salivary protein putrefaction and malodor production. Quintessence Int. 2006;37(8):653–8.

Sterer N, Nuas S, Mizrahi B, Goldenberg C, Weiss EI, Domb A, Davidi MP. Oral malodor reduction by a palatal mucoadhesive tablet containing herbal formulation. J Dent. 2008;36(7):535–9.

Printed in the United States
by Baker & Taylor Publisher Services